THE GRIM
REAPER
WREAKING HAVOC
SINCE 2019

COVID-19

DR. PRASANNAJEET PRAMOD NIKAM

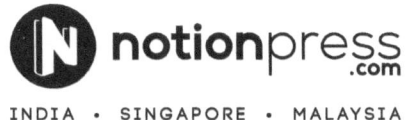

INDIA · SINGAPORE · MALAYSIA

Notion Press Media Pvt Ltd

No. 50, Chettiyar Agaram Main Road,
Vanagaram, Chennai, Tamil Nadu – 600 095

First Published by Notion Press 2021
Copyright © Dr. Prasannajeet Pramod Nikam 2021
All Rights Reserved.

ISBN 978-1-63940-395-0

CONTENTS

1 | ACKNOWLEDGEMENT

I would like to express my sincere gratitude to my parents, Mr.Pramod Nikam and Mrs.Ulhasini Nikam for their unconditional love, constant support and belief in me irrespective of my endeavor. I never got a chance to thank my mummy and pappa for their upbringing and for all the hardships and difficult times they faced while fulfilling each and every single tantrum of me. I know "thank you" is a very small word which would fail to address their sacrifice. So I dedicate this book to my Pappa and Mummy as a big yet too small "Thank-You" for making me what I am today. Also, a big thank you to my younger sister Mayuri for forgiving me for not mentioning her in the acknowledgement of my first book "**Physiotherapy in COVID-19: Role & Scope of PT in corona pandemic.**"

A big thank you to Hon'ble Chatrapati.Shri.Udayanraje Bhosale Ji; Member of Parliament (MP); for his availability in need and for being the biggest pillar of support for the people of Satara.

It takes me immense joy to express my deepest gratitude for Hon'ble Chatrapati Shri Shivendra Singh Raje Bhosale Ji; Member of Legislative Assembly (MLA), for showing concern about knowing minor details of the book.

I am very much indebted to Hon'ble. Jaykumar Gore Ji;Member of Legislative Assembly (MLA), for generously accepting my request to express his views about the book.

I extend my gratitude to Dr.Suresh Bhosale Ji; Chancellor; Krishna Institute of Medical Sciences "Deemed To Be University", Karad; for being a role model and inspiration to many people like me who want to make their "karma-bhoomi" proud!

I am eternally grateful to Dr.Atul BhosaleJi;Hon'ble Chairman; Krishna Sahakari Bank; for always being there for me inspite of his extremely tight schedule. Thank you for always managing to respond to my help calls!

I find myself extremely lucky to have the guidance and support of Mr.Vinayak Bhosale Ji; Member of Board of Management; Krishna Institute of Medical Sciences deemed to be University,Karad.

My deepest gratitude to Dr.Pravin Shingare Ji; Hon'ble Pro-Chancellor,Krishna Institute of Medical Sciences "Deemed To Be University", Karad; for his unconditional support and constant motivation. I thank you sir for the belief you have shown in me.

It would just be unfair by all means if I forget to express my extreme thankfulness to Dr.Dinesh Agarwal Sir; Additional Director of Research, Krishna Institute of Medical Sciences "Deemed to be University", for instilling the qualities of a good researcher in me. I thank you from the bottom of my heart for developing interest for research in me.

My heartfelt gratefulness to Mrs.Nishriin Parikh Ji; International Body Builders Federation(IBBF) International Physique Athlete and Fitness model and Celebrity; for putting the same energy and enthusiasm she puts on stage while representing India; while writing the testimonial for this book. I thank you mam for being so kind and generous to give your valuable thoughts to this book!

A big shout out to my brother Mr.Nikhil Chindak; International Roller Skater; member of the Roller skating World Cup winning Indian team; one of the strongest pillars of my life for always being there for me.

I would be failing in my duties if I didn't mention my Alma matter, Krishna College of Physiotherapy, Karad for providing me the opportunity to contribute my share towards the service to mankind. I thank each and every patient from "COVID-19 Care Centre" of

Krishna Hospital and Medical Research Centre for their co-operation and patience which played a very crucial role in the conduction of various research projects.

Special thanks to all the staff at Notionpress Publications for their constant support throughout the publication process. Right from designing the cover till marketing the book; the entire process felt like a cake-walk with you all.

And last but not the least, Special thanks to Dr.Aishwarya Bulbule for always being my first proof-reader, critic, editor and most important of all – My energy ! My sincere apologies if I have forgot to mention anyone. I would like to appreciate direct as well as indirect support of all my colleagues and friends whose contributions helped me in my journey.

2 | FOREWORD

The main aim to publish this book in the chronological stages of COVID-19, since its first cycle till now when we are facing adverse effects of second cycle and marching towards cure and care through vaccination.

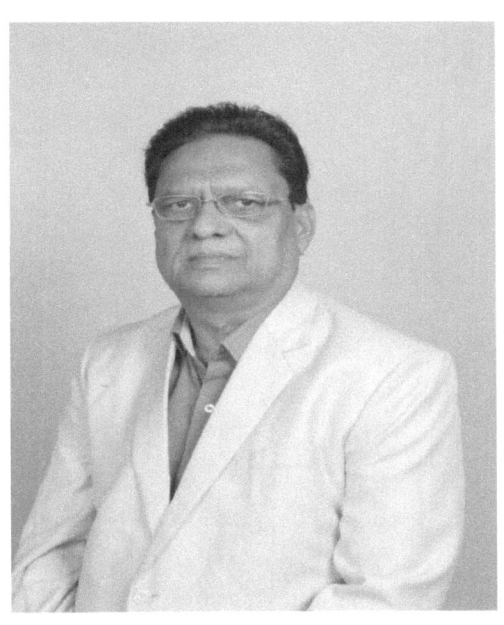

The loss occurred during these phases upon human being in the form of illness, loss of livelihood, monetary loss and ultimately mortality and morbidity which cannot be anticipated in the perspective of country in particular and world as a whole and post-covid problems which are being affect the society is another factor.The research could be able to demonstrate few solutions as a protocol for livelihood and also other preventive measures from throughout the world but as research is a never ending process therefore, it is too early to mention about the future which can be faced by the society.In the present context this book is well organized in the form of different chapters, those cover all phases of the COVID-19 and upto post-covid preventive measures.

I wish that the content of the book shall be highly appreciated by the society by adopting various practices as contained in the book in their routine life.

Dr.D.K.Agarwal

Additional Director of Research

Krishna Institute of Medical Sciences "Deemed To be University"

Testimonials

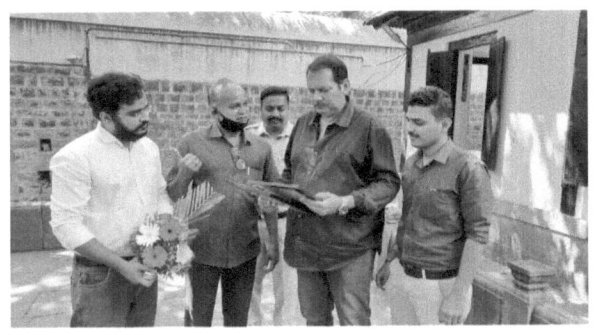

"COVID-19 pandemic is the unanswered question rooting in the society. It has not spared any fragment of the society from its vicious grip of claws. People are suffering, economies are collapsing and countries are shutting down amidst this pandemic. In such a holocaust, where in even temples of gods are closed; it is the medical healthcare professionals who are working at the frontline day and night, combating against the COVID-19 virus.

Dr.Prasannajeet's initiation to provide a guide which would help the people during such difficult times is very much appreciable. He has done a splendid job by trying to incorporate the necessary factual information which needs to be delivered, not only to the people of this country, but to the people located all over the globe. And I am confident that this book will do its part in spreading awareness and be the ultimate torch of enlightment and hope in everyone's lives!

Wishing you all the success!

Regards."

Hon'ble Shri. Chatrapati Udayanraje Bhosale Ji

Member of Parliament (MP)

Satara Constituency

Testimonials

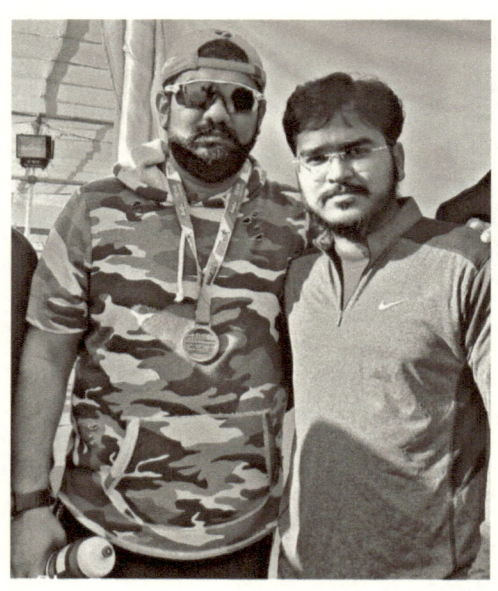

"Role of Physiotherapists is very distinguished in managing the crisis along with other health care professionals. I am well acquainted about physiotherapy as I myself have needed it occasionally. And I would like to thank all of the health care professionals today for your hard work, thoughtfulness, and commitment during this challenging time. Among the heroes who have emerged from this crisis are the health care professionals who have risked their own health to serve their patients. The nation is indebted to you.

Dr.Prasannajeet being a extremely talented sports physiotherapist; we have met quite a few times before during various marathon events organized all over Satara district, where he led a team of physiotherapists as "medical care unit". Besides being a physiotherapist, he is an excellent artist and writer. I am sure that this book; being written by such eminent hands, will continue to serve its noble intentions and will prove to be rejuvenating in the lives of COVID-19 affected people.

Much power to you and your book!

Regards."

Hon'ble Chatrapati Shri. Shivendra Singh Raje Bhosale Ji

Member of Legislative Assembly (MLA)

Testimonials

I am delighted to write this testimonial for Dr.Prasannajeet's upcoming book titled **"COVID-19: The Grim Reaper wreaking havoc since 2019".** In an age where COVID-19 has devastated the core of our mother earth, it is very crucial to stay updated about the course of the disease. But seeing the huge ocean of resources available online as well as offline, the originality of the information becomes a matter of debate. Dr.Prasannajeet has beautifully explained about all the doubts and queries related to COVID-19 in a very sophisticated manner. It contains facts supported with scientific literature arranged in a manner easily comprehendible by layman. I hope this book reaches to every corner of the globe and helps to spread awareness and eradicate perplexity which prevails in the society about COVID-19!

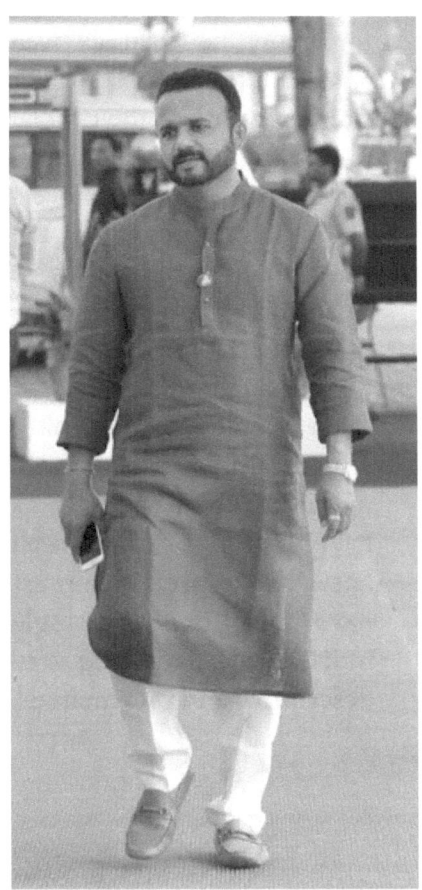

My very best wishes for all of your future endeavors!

Regards.

Hon'ble. Jaykumar Gore Ji

Member of Legislative Assembly (MLA)

Maan-Khataav Constituency

Testimonials

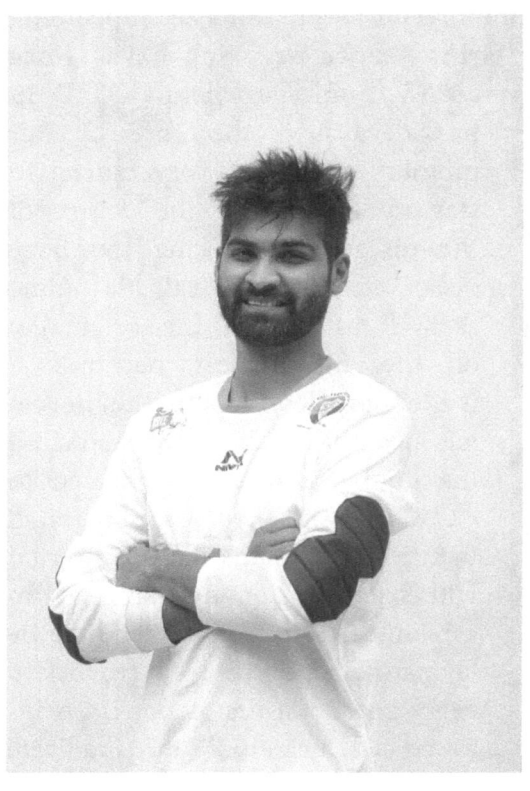

"I know Dr.Prasannajeet since his post-graduation days. He has been there for many national as well as international roller skating events as the official physiotherapist. Politeness, persistence and never-giving up attitude are the three qualities of him which I admire the most. The book is just fantastic. Easy to understand even for those people who don't have a medical field background. All FAQ's about COVID-19 have been very well answered by him. It's a must have book for every single individual. It is indeed very descriptive and informative!

May you continue this noble job brother!

Lots of love."

Mr. Nikhil Chindak

Team Member of World-Cup Winning Indian Roller Skating Team

Testimonials

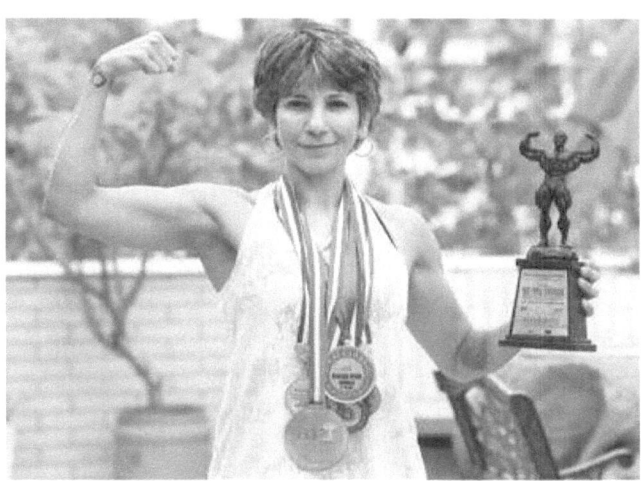

To all the doctors out there; I would like to take up this opportunity to express how grateful I am for your day and night hard work and dedicated service to mankind. Just like others, this dreadful pandemic has taken on you all too, but it is this commitment to your oath and sacrifice of your life for the healing of the sick which stands in between the COVID-19 virus and we people. Words won't be enough to express what you all mean to this nation and to the entire world! Dr.Prasannajeet has done his bit for the society by extending the knowledge in the form of scientific literature simplified for the easy comprehension of the layman. His book "The Grim Reaper Wreaking Havoc since 2019: COVID-19" is an excellent source of all the guidelines, information, facts and scientific details related to COVID-19. It is informative to the core and will definitely prove to be the guiding light for the needy!

I wish him all the best and hope that he continues this splendid job forever!

Mrs.Nishriin Parikh

International Physique Athlete

54 yrs old Fitness model, GladRags Mrs India finalist

GNC Ambassador and founder of Yogasstrength.

3 | PREFACE

COVID-19 pandemic still continues to be the prime concern for the health-care system throughout the world. While some of the developed super-powers of the world are still struggling in combating and stopping the exponentially growing cases of COVID-19 cases, India has been able to implement damage control to some extent. The major credit goes to the extremely efficient health care system of our nation. In spite of facing multiple challenges like recalcitrant public, unavailability of a potent vaccine, limited infrastructure and economic instability secondary to lockdowns, India has emerged strong and continues to march on the path towards defeating this novel corona virus. The healthcare professionals have been rightly addressed as "Frontline COVID-19 heroes" by our beloved honorable Prime Minister Shri.Narendra Modi ji. It is the constant relentless efforts of doctors, nurses, paramedics, sanitation department and all other supporting staff that have saved millions of lives and led to the consolidation of the path of recovery. Physiotherapists are one among these heroes who are striving hard for the ultimate betterment of COVID-19 survivors.

I, being a physiotherapist myself, have worked in Intensive Care Unit named "COVID-19 Care Centre" of Krishna Institute of Medical Sciences Deemed to be University, Karad. Six to eight hours of shifts for one entire week followed by one week of mandatory quarantine period was the schedule which is still being followed. At first, I was very much elated to be a small contributor in helping and managing COVID-19 affected people. But as days passed by and as the number of positive cases started increasing exponentially, I experienced a strange discomfort. This discomfort wasn't physical. It wasn't even describable. It was just a vague feeling of incompleteness. I felt there is something lacking from my side which I owe to those bed-ridden patients. I felt I owe more than just positioning them on ICU water-beds. I felt I owe more than just asking them to repeat breathing exercises thrice a day. I felt I owed them a much better life in spite of trying my level best. This feeling of indebtedness led me towards the path of finding the missing piece of the puzzle. This is what acted like a driving force for finding the lacunae in existing scarce literature on physiotherapy in COVID-19.

I started reading articles about the current recent advances for managing a COVID-19 patient in ICU. Standard recommendations had been set by some researchers on stage wise indication for physiotherapy in such patients. While working closely with COVID-19 patients, I observed that these recommendations can't be generalized. Post-COVID-19 rehabilitation needed to be given equal importance like treating COVID-19 itself. I identified the less focused areas like combination exercises for physical rehabilitation, daily routine modifications to be adapted by patients to ensure psychological well being, guidelines to ensure safety for the physiotherapists, alternative & cost-efficient devices for cardio-pulmonary rehabilitation and holistic treatment approach by utilizing other supportive therapies; which lacked sufficient physiotherapeutic literature. And thus, I decided to start the pavement of my "dream-project".

Writing every single word of this book gave me euphoria as it was one of my biggest dreams to express my thoughts and feelings about my profession in front of the world. I believe this book is a direct dialogue between me and my fellow physiotherapist, a small gesture to unleash the hidden potential and highlight multiple roles played by these "unsung heroes"! I hope this book will help the budding physiotherapists to develop a research-oriented perspective in order to improve their skills as well as benefit the patients.

4 | MYTHS DEBUNKED...FACTS EXPLAINED

COVID-19 is undoubtedly the greatest teacher who has taught us some of the biggest lessons of life since 2019. A lot of stir up is going on in the society between myths and facts related to COVID-19. People are facing perplexity in taking simple decisions in their day to day life due to the total mix-up of news and information related to this dreadful disease. One of the many reasons behind writing this book is to help reduce the turmoil prevailing amongst people related to this disease. At present, there is no prediction available which would conclusively comment on how long this pandemic will extend. So, the only way by which we can directly contribute towards constraining the spread of this perilous virus is by being the spreader of facts. Today; when everyone is well versed with the physical health aspect of this disease, it is the need of the hour to focus on the psychosocial implications of the pandemic. People need to understand that along with physical rehabilitation it is also the psychological support which is there to offer to the needy during these difficult times.

Commercialization of the health care services is going on full-fledged in the society. The sacred oath of Hippocrates is losing its value somewhere down the line. Practicing medicine has become more of a money-mining business than life-saving noble profession which it used to be. This pandemic has overshadowed the humanitarian side and revealed the cruel face of selfishness!

This book is intended to help people identify the hidden traps along their road. The sole purpose is to provide a guide which will initiate the eradication of all the pessimism, perplexity, callousness and trepidation from the minds of the people. This book carries the ultimate goal to provide the people with patronage which will be their vital energy source and driving force in this grueling war against COVID-19!

People are walking through a long, dark tunnel of COVID-19. While walking they are facing challenges like shortage of oxygen, misleading traps of perplexity and stigmas, etc. Some of the individuals who are not receiving the support from their very own bodies are losing the race midway. The race is for life! With the huge COVID-19 monster chasing us, we have to remember that our only chance to outrun the virus is by following the safety and precautionary norms laid down by the government. There is light at the end of the tunnel, for sure! All we need is a guide to the path which will take us to that mother earth which will be thriving in harmony…free of COVID-19!

5 | NE HAO, WO SHI COVID 19!

(Hello, I am COVID-19!)

To,

The Human Beings.

Hello Humans! It's been nearly 2 years since we first met. But, still I am just an acquaintance to you. You don't know much about me. So here I am to tell you my story in my words. I was born in the month of November 2019 in Wuhan, China. Before that I was jailed to live only in animals. I have been there since centuries. I used to see you people through the eyes of the animals. You seemed so happy, enjoying life with friends, having family dinners on weekends, exploring various places and having a wonderful life! I envied you and was so jealous of your world filled with peace and joy. But one day; when I got up from my sleep, I noticed I was no longer inside the body of an animal. I wondered how come I got shifted to this new place. I was very happy with my new house though. But my owner didn't appear to enjoy my company. As I was out of jail after so many centuries, I started growing stress-free. I roamed in my big house everywhere. And finally got cozy in the **"lungs"** room. Here, I met my wife and we had so many children. As our little family got expanded, we had no space to accommodate. So, we started exploring other rooms of my new house and in this way we took over the control of the entire house.

Then one fine day, my new owner decided to meet up with his friends. This was our chance to buy more estate for our exponentially expanding family. Suddenly we were sucked in by a strong vacuum through a tunnel (bronchus, nasopharynx and oropharynx) and in no time we were out in the open world! It was not less than a roller-coaster ride for us! Once we were out, we saw there were many houses in the world, ready to be infected by us. It was a world full of food and shelter for us. So we got spread to other houses. Some of our new owners travelled out to other countries, which helped me expand nationally and globally. And on 11th March 2020; it was officially declared by the World Health Organization (WHO) that we had captured the entire earth.

Everything was going good when suddenly; when I was about to left my house to enter other houses, I found out that the door of the tunnel was closed. In spite of several attempts, I was not able to open or break it. They say it was made up of "N-95 Mask". So I remained trapped inside my own house. But some of my friends said their tunnels were closed with "normal cloth mask" which were easy to break unlike the "N-95 mask door". Also people stopped meeting each other and preferred staying inside their own house. This was a red-alert for us as many of my friends were dying by staying trapped inside their respective houses. The vaccine came as a "disaster" for us shattering our dreams of conquering the world.

But, all thanks to some **"COVIDIOTS"** we managed to continue our legacy till date. Now I have become a part of your life. There is hardly any human left on the planet who has not heard my name. There is hardly anyone who has not lost his family member or closed one's to me. Today I am the headline of each and every newspaper. I am the breaking news on each and every news channel. I am the one who has put a "full stop" to the entire world. I am the one who has inflicted physical, mental, economical and social hardships on you people. All thanks to your "karma" I am still thriving on this beautiful planet spreading misery, fear, misunderstandings and death.

I am "**The Grim Reaper Wreaking Havoc since 2019**".

Unwillingly Yours,

COVID-19.

6 | WELCOME TO THE COVID-19 ERA!

The novel corona virus which is also called as "Wuhan virus" has changed the dynamics of how things used to be. The awful disease has led to the shutdown of the entire globe. Killing millions of people, shattering billions of families and bringing the economies to the ruin; the outbreak of this pandemic has clearly proved what irresponsible behavior of humans can do to the balance of the eco-system. This pandemic has clearly dictated its terms that if you go against the nature, you will have to face the wrath of it. The ongoing critical period is a mirror reflection of how we treated animals, birds, fishes and all other components of the ecosystem. Human beings captivate animals and birds by keeping them in cages simply to fulfill their desire of entertainment. But now the same karma has been acting upon human fate. We have been forced to be confined within our four walled cage called "home" whereas animals are roaming the streets freely. This is the biggest and worst damage which we have inflicted upon ourselves in the history of mankind.

Adaptation is one of the human instincts which make survival in extremes of conditions possible. Currently when breathing air is nothing less than inhaling poison, the fittest are surviving where as the weak are falling prey to the claws of this dreadful disease. We are like animals today trapped in our own house, unable to see each other's faces without mask. Today, the highest level of intimacy is to able to see each other through a glass-wall partition. A mother can't even be the receiver of the sheer happiness of holding her newborn baby after giving birth if she is known case of COVID-19.

It is very rightly said – "Change is the only permanent thing in this world". The late 2019 has triggered another change in ways which were unimaginable by human-brains a few years back. Social-distancing, hygienic practices and increased health concerns are the factors which have modified our way of life. This is going to go a long way. In others words this is the new "normal" lifestyle. Apart from having physical consequences, the infestation of this disease has left deep psychological consequences on the society. People are under constant threat of acquiring the disease (coronaphobia) which is affecting their inter-personal relationships. Post-COVID Stress Disorder as well as Post-COVID Syndrome are the relatively newer mental health concerns which have been bothering a significant proportion of the population all over the globe. Economies are in the toilet and the percentage of unemployment is at the peak.

Additionally, there is no great success in containing the COVID-19 cases in spite of mass vaccination drive initiated by the governments of various countries. Initially the efficacy of the vaccines in stopping the corona virus was very less. Still there is no certainty about the time-gap to be kept between the first dose and the second dose of the vaccine. The constantly mutating strains of the COVID-19 virus are reducing the spectrum of effect of various vaccines which have been developed. Many nations across the globe who are having good international ties with India have been helping us with whatever means possible.

The ultimate option of attaining "**herd immunity**" is also not viable anymore as the scientists have failed to calculate the "**herd threshold level**" which has been attributed to the "highly unstable morphology" of the novel coronavirus. The latest of the strain which has been identified as "**B.1.617**". This double mutant strain is a hybrid of two variants namely **L452R** and **E484Q**. Out of the two core mutations, the E484Q is very similar to the E484K which is exclusively found in the South African and Brazilian variants. The E484K mutation is also called as the "**escape mutation**" as it strengthens the virus by enabling the SARS-CoV-2 to escape the encounter with monoclonal antibodies. This is the primary reason why vaccines have been proving ineffective or less potent in curbing the spread of the virus. This variant has been named "most transmissible variant" of COVID-19. It is the strain which has infected majority of people in India; specifically Maharashtra and is also responsible for the high death toll in the second wave of the pandemic.

Apart from all the direct as well indirect contributing factors responsible for the spread of COVID-19; the main factor which is proving to be the ultimate culprit for increased agitation in the society is the "unawareness". Believing myths or false alarms related to COVID-19 is just making the condition worse amongst the crowd. It is the need of the hour to formulate some strict protocols for extended medical services. The government needs to focus on establishing regional consolidated pathways of information release and distribution in order to create less confusion among the masses regarding the credibility or authenticity of the news. Appropriate channeling of the resources through government regulated authorities can help to curb black marketing of the essential commodities. In order to avoid the financial exploitation going on by the private hospitals, medical and surgical supply stores, etc. standardization of prices has to be done from time to time by the respective government authorities. Implementation of regular surprise audits; to check any illegal stocking of essential commodities to create false shortage in order to inflate the prices, should be done right from the rural level itself.

This COVID-19 pandemic is a live telecast of how difficult it can get to dream to live a normal life. It is a display of the fact that how priceless it is to even be able to just survive each day and look up to the rise of the other. It is a constant reminder to the entire human race about how lucky were we to be able to breathe in fresh air. But it's very rightly said "you don't realize the value of anything until you lose it for good". Now, people have started realizing the value of possessing a healthy body. The importance of workout in order to maintain an optimal fitness level has been constantly highlighted as a crucial initiative during this pandemic. People have never been so conscious about their diet, personal hygiene, health monitoring as well as social responsibilities as they are in these difficult times.

Before the pandemic, we were physically close but emotionally miles from each other. During COVID-19 pandemic, we might be miles from each other physically, but the circumstances have made us grow closer to each other emotionally. It's ironic how social-distancing has brought us more close emotionally!

7 | AFTER(COVID-19)LIFE

Physical, Social & Mental Challenges of a COVID-19 Survivor

The society is witnessing a change since the onset of this pandemic. Change in terms of lifestyle, human behavior, quality of life, economy etc. The change can be identified at various levels. Starting from individual level till the national or global level, the corona crisis has changed the way things used to be. According to experts, this is our modified lifestyle and it is mandatory that we adopt and improvise ourselves accordingly.

But, various factors are responsible for determining an individual's ability to adopt and adjust to this modified lifestyle. Physical, mental as well as social aspects are the chief determinants which influence the survival instinct of an individual. All the three mentioned aspects need to be in perfect balance for a human being to endure any disaster that changes his quality of life.

A positive Rapid Antigen Test or RT-PCR Test result is the point at which change starts in an individual's life. At times, it's just the mere presence of one of the symptoms in an individual which agitates him/her along with the entire family. It is not only the person who is affected; it is a blow to the entire family. Given the prevailing situation and the lack of adequate sturdy literature on COVID-19 and its prognosis, the emotional instability is evident to kick in. The various contributory factors like financial status, availability of health resources, area of residence, socio-economic status etc just add in to the existing chaos. Thus, it becomes very crucial for a physiotherapist to have a deep insight in all aspects of life as it helps him to understand the rehabilitative demands of the patient.

The lockdown, loss of social life, unemployment and mortality due to COVID-19 are the main reasons for the wave of psychological disturbance in the population. According to scientists deterioration of mental health can start as a mere apprehension or fear for the novel corona virus disease. This irrational fear has been termed as "Coronaphobia". Coronaphobia have been defined by the scientists as "an excessive triggered response of fear of contracting the virus causing COVID-19, leading to accompanied excessive concern over physiological symptoms, significant stress about personal and occupational loss, increased reassurance and safety seeking behaviors, and avoidance of public places and situations, causing marked impairment in daily life functioning".

Quality of Life of a COVID-19 Survivor

In current scenario, getting beds with Oxygen and/or ventilator support is a very difficult task. People are being denied admission in hospitals as the managements are not having adequate oxygen supplies And even if one manages to get admitted, the symptoms and the progression of the disease make it more difficult. Presence of other co morbidities or belonging to the vulnerable age group determine the fate of the patient. If the patient succumbs to ventilator support, then the chances of developing anxiety and depression get elevated considerably. Especially if he/she lacks a proper familial support. Thus, mental health conditioning becomes of prime importance right from the pre-ICU or ICU stage itself.

Stage-wise Contributor for Deterioration of Mental Status in COVID-19 Patients

A COVID-19 patient has to battle many mental catastrophic battles in addition to the fight against physical progressively aggravating symptoms. Right from the day when he is tested positive until he is discharged and returns home, there are many factors which directly as well as indirectly try to bring down a COVID-19 survivor emotionally and mentally. We never know which part of our behavior might be contributing to the mental degradation or breakdown of a COVID-19 survivor. A COVID-19 patient goes through a series of stages till his complete recovery. The stages are as follows-

1. Active infection stage

2. General Hospitalization stage

3. Intensive Care Unit (ICU) stage

4. Rehabilitation stage

5. Recovery stage

6. Post-recovery stage/Return to pre-morbid stage

1. *Active Infection Stage*

Active infection stage is the duration from diagnosis till hospital admission for acute stay. If a person is having any of the COVID-19 symptoms or if he has been recently in close contact with a COVID-19 positive person, then ideally he should go for Rapid antigen test or RT-PCR test. If the tests come positive, then it becomes crucial to plan the proceedings. This has to be done by anticipating consequences and trusting your instincts. This is only possible when you have a complete understanding of your own body. To understand this more clearly, we have to consider the following scenarios which might arise in case of active infection stage.

Scenario 1 – If a person is positive, but is asymptomatic i.e. he doesn't have any symptoms of the disease; then he should prefer isolating himself at home.

Scenario 2 – If a person is positive and having mild symptoms

Scenario 3 – If a person is positive and having moderate to severe symptoms

Scenario 4 – If a person is negative and still having some symptoms; then ideally he should go for a re-test. Such false positive or false negative results might arise due to other inflammatory conditions also. So, on the basis of the above scenarios appropriate decisions have to be made whether a person inevitably needs to be admitted to a acute hospital setting.

Challenges

A positive Rapid Antigen Test or RT-PCR is the trigger for panic, anxiety or depression in patients. And this is passively transferred to the entire family. Some individuals don't proceed to hospital admission simply due to the fear of facing social rejection. This perception of derogatory response is more profoundly felt by sensitive people or extroverts. The sudden change in people's point of view towards self is a hard thing to accept especially for the weak minded. You never know how your unkind words or disparaging deeds might have a negative effect on people with COVID-19.

2. General Hospitalization Stage

If the symptoms of a COVID-19 positive patient get aggravated (moderate to severe), then he may need to be shifted to a acute hospital setting. This is usually done to manage aggravated symptoms like breathlessness or difficulty in breathing, vomiting, chest pain etc. Usually individuals with co morbidities like asthma, diabetes, chronic renal failure, etc. face rapid progression of the symptoms. This ultimately leads to involvement of various parts of the body which produces the associated symptom thus making it mandatory to transfer the patient to hospital for further treatment.

Challenges

The existing coronaphobia just amplifies the panic which a patient has already acquired through various factors like news, false messages being circulated on social medias, death of someone close etc.

3. Intensive Care Unit (ICU) Stage

This stage is the most crucial of all stages as the fate of the patient relies heavily on his/her prognosis during the overall intensive care unit stay. The overall high mortality of COVID-19 patients can be attributed to the unpredictable course a patient can take during his ICU stay. Multiple factors might contribute to the same like-

- Presence of Co morbid conditions.
- Delay in hospitalization.
- Hospital acquired infections.
- Multi-organ failure.
- Acute Respiratory Distress Syndrome (ARDS).
- Pneumonia.
- Development of blood clots ultimately leading to thrombus or emboli.
- Septicemia secondary to bed-sores.

4. Rehabilitation Stage

This is the stage where in the patient is out of the associated complications and has been able to maintain his vitals without any supporting devices like ventilator or NIV masks. In case of COVID-19; a patient is said to be stable if he/she is able to maintain SPO_2 level of **95%**≤without any external support & if he/she has not shown any of the symptoms of COVID-19 in the past 3 days.

5. Recovery Stage

Recovery stage commences once the patient gets adapted to the rehabilitation process. Physical Therapy has to be done on a regular basis. Graded exercises for cardiopulmonary endurance along with muscular strengthening should be initiated and gradually progressed to active assisted and resisted exercises.

6. Post-recovery Stage/Return to Pre-morbid Stage

Following complete physical therapy rehabilitation period, the individual is said to be physically fit if he/she is able to perform some of the physical fitness assessment tests like 6-min walk test, Treadmill stress test etc.

8 | TIMELINE OF COVID-19 MUTATIONS

Emergence of Various Strains Throughout the Course of the Pandemic

COVID-19 has been the biggest challenge since the late 2019. Although vaccines have been developed to curb the further spread of the pandemic and to achieve "herd-immunity", controlling the mortality rate still appears to be a uphill task. The SARS-CoV-2 virus has undergone mutations resulting in different variants scattered all over the globe. It is important to know a bit about the history of evolution of this virus into the "big-bull" which it has become today!

A US government interagency group has developed a variant classification scheme that categorizes different SARS-CoV-2 variants into three main classes. The classes are as follows:

1. **Variant of Interest**

2. **Variant of Concern**

3. **Variant of High Consequence**

1. Variant of Interest (VOI)

These variants usually contain a special genetic marker which is already known to cause-

1. Changes to the receptor binding sites making the adherence of the virus to human host cells comparatively easier.

2. Reduction in the neutralization effect of antibodies generated by previous exposure to infection or those acquired through vaccination.

3. Reduction in the efficacy of various treatment approaches.

4. High increase in transmissibility or disease severity.

B.1.525, B.1.526, B.1.526.1, B.1.617, B.1.617.1, B.1.617.2, B.1.617.3 and **P.2** are the examples of variants of interest.

All of the above mentioned variants have one mutation in common which is known as "**D614G**". This is the mutation which was seen in Europe and later circulated in U.S.A.

2. *Variant of Concern (VOC)*

Variant of Concern (VOC) have all the attributes of Variant of Interest (VOI) and additionally it has relatively higher hospitalization and death rates as well as lower detection rates on various diagnostic tests.

B.1.1.7, B.1.351, B.1.427, B.1.429 and **P.1** are the variants belonging to the VOC class.

3. *Variants of High Consequence (VOHC)*

A Variant of High Consequence (VHC) has all the attributes of Variants of Interest (VOI) and Variant of Concern (VOC) and additionally it has the highest mortality as well as hospitalization rates. This class contains the most severe variant of SARS-CoV-2. Currently, there are no variants which have been included in this class.

SARS-CoV-2 emerged in Wuhan, China in November 2019. Later this virus underwent mutation in terms of **D614G** substitution in the late January or early February 2020. And this circulated in the major parts of the world covering the entire globe by June 2020. It was found out through several research studies that the variant **D614G** mutation was more infective and transmissible as compared to the original **SARS-CoV-2** found in China, but had no serious mortality or hospitalization levels.

A new variant, named as "**cluster 5**" was then reported from the North Jutland of Denmark. The mutations in this particular variant were not known or mentioned previously. It was found out later that this variant had less transmission capacity.

The United Kingdom reported a new variant **SARS-CoV-2 VOC 2020 12/01**. Although its origin is unclear, it was believed to come from South East England and by 26th December it had spread in the entire United Kingdom. By 30th December the VOC 2020 12/01 variant had spread all over the globe affecting countries/territories/areas.

Later South Africa reported cases of rapidly spreading new strain of SARS-CoV-2 which was named as **501Y.V2.** As of the data received on 30th December, the predominant **501Y.V2**variant from South Africa was reported in four more countries across the globe.

Factors Influencing Global Variations in COVID-19 Cases

Uneven distribution of COVID-19 cases across the globe triggered the research studies to investigate the various factors responsible for global variations in the COVID-19 cases. According to a study by Hammad et al. (2020); the spread of COVID-19 depend on the following factors-

1. Population Characteristics

2. Environmental and Geographic factors

3. Healthcare policy

4. Virus related Factors: Strain of the virus

1. Population Characteristics

It includes various sub-factors like Age, sex, genetic makeup, social lifestyle factors, population density and number of elder care facilities.

2. Environmental & Geographic Factors

It includes factors like pollution levels, type of climate, 5G internet communication, travel rate etc.

3. Healthcare Policy

It consists of various factors like under-reporting of statistics, timely response of governments, national policy of BCG vaccination, Employment and scale of diagnostic testing, implementation of social distancing norms and physical resources and healthcare workforce.

4. Virus Related Factors: Strain of the Virus

Strain of the prevailing virus can prove to be the biggest of the factors responsible for regional variations in COVID-19 cases.

9 | BREAK THE(MONEY) CHAIN!

How not to Fall Prey to Money Extradition During this Pandemic?

As 2021 is advancing, we are witnessing a surge in the number of COVID-19 cases in India. The new mutated strains of the corona virus are hitting hard specially in this stage which is believed to be the second wave of this dreadful pandemic. It has been declared that witnessing the current rate of spread of the pandemic, India is bound to hit the third wave in October or November month of 2021.

So, in order to create awareness among the society about the ongoing malpractices and to ensure that we don't fall in such trap; the **"BREAK THE CHAIN"** guideline has been formulated. Each letter of the pneumonic stands for single guideline by following which we can ensure that we do not fall prey to unnecessary financial burdening.It consists of 13 steps to be followed by all of us during this pandemic to make sure that no one falls prey to the money-minting business which has been going on nowadays.

Beware of Fraudulent People

Financial exploitation is the key factor which is prevailing in society on a larger extent. Right from getting bed till getting space for the final rites of a COVID-19 patient in crematorium, families of the patients are getting scammed by fraudsters. Extra money is being forced on the families of COVID-19 patients for allowance of basic things like medicines, O_2 cylinders, antibiotics, etc. There are some unethical individuals with no humanity who are feeding off the helplessness of the COVID-19 patients as well as their families. But it can be limited if each and every individual decides to contribute his/her bit towards awareness about the unethical practices going on in the society.

Reliability of Source

The first and foremost step is to depend on reliable sources for hospital admission. Many instances have been reported wherein the family of the patient has been deceived by fraudsters who claim to make available bed in a particular hospital. They ask for advance money which is usually 2–3 times that of normal charges. Out of desperation, families of patients hastily pay out all the money without authenticating the source of help and thus ultimately become a victim of financial exploitation.

Ensure Online Security

The government is trying to expand the outreach of medical facilities by digitalizing health care services. The goal is to ensure that there is no discrimination in terms of availability of basic medical care facilities. But, as it's rightly said that each coin has two sides; same saying holds true for the digitalization of the health care services. Especially during such critical COVID-19 times where each and everyone is struggling to seek the medical attention at any cost, there are high chances that people might be victims of increasing cyber crimes and cyber frauds.

Avoid Advance Payments

Hospitalization is the stepping stone for the commencement of financial crisis especially for the lower and middle socioeconomic classes of the society. Individuals with very less or no backup of medical insurances, health cover or saving funds find it extremely difficult to manage huge amount in a relatively shorter period of time.

In such circumstances of scarce financial resources one should plan it very well to avoid facing financial insufficiencies. There are reported instances in New Delhi where people have been scammed by unknown fraudsters by telling to deposit advance money to some account for oxygen tank delivery.

Keep Important Contact Details Handy

It has been observed that in spite of availability of certain resources, their access to the needy is blocked due to the absence of appropriate contact method. Most people are not able to establish a contact with the source of help and thus remain unreached. So, list of all hospitals, oxygen suppliers, ambulance service providers, pharmacists, blood banks, plasma banks, etc should be made by the respective mayor of town and it should be circulated by authenticating it with government seal or letterhead. By this way, people will stop believing fake news and posts and thus will in turn help to reduce the pre-existing chaos.

Try not to Panic

Amidst the ruckus which has been going on, a general tendency of believing in any news feed or circular from unauthenticated sources is seen among the people. Various fake news and messages are being circulated. It is the responsibility of each and every one of us to believe only on information from a scientific or government source. Especially the medical professionals and health-care workers have to take the lead in erasing the misconceptions and false beliefs related to COVID-19 prevailing in the society. This can be done by creating discussion forums in every colony or every society. The respective medical or health care professional can control the posts, messages, important links etc in the group.

Help the Needy

The upper class people are fleeing this country as they no longer feel safe in our country. Celebrities are going to exotic destinations for spending holidays when people are gasping for air and dying in the country. While a few bunch of financially privileged people are coming forward and doing their bit to help the less privileged people. May it be donating to the PM Relief Fund or may it be providing free food for the healthcare professionals; responsible people are doing their bit in tackling COVID-19.

Ethical Practice

Being medicos, we are ethically and professionally bound by the Hippocrates's Oath. We have to ensure ethical practice at all times. Especially during these pandemic times where saving people's lives has been taken up as a life-mission by some noble people, there are also a group of people trying to take advantage of helplessness of the people. Free consultations are being given online by some doctors. There are some NGO's distributing food, water, clothes, medicines, O_2 cylinders etc. Existence of such angel souls is proving that humanity is still alive in this world and will help us swim across this ocean of disaster.

Complaint against Malpractices

Stop being a mute spectator and start reporting and protesting against any unethical practices like over-charging, adulteration, misleading information, false alarms etc. By being vigilante you can be the pioneer in establishing peace and harmony in the presently agitated society.

Humanity

The circumstances are so vicious nowadays that people are literally gasping for oxygen. Families are undergoing through a lot of torment in order to secure a bed for their dying member. Without having food and water for whole day; people are standing in mile long Queue's in scorching heat just to be lucky enough to get a single vial of remdesivir or tocilizumab.There are a few people who are working days and night's altogether to serve the one's in need.

Awareness

Try to spread awareness from the root level. Do your bit to contribute to a noble cause of eradicating the darkness of misbelieves and perplexity. Use whatever means available to start a awareness campaign. Start it alone and people with noble cause will join you along the way.

Insist for Basic Rights

Nelson Mandela has very rightly said, "To deny people their basic rights is to challenge their very humanity." Government is trying their level best to make sure that no one gets left out from receiving the benefits of various relief schemes implemented at various levels. But, it is also our duty to be aware about our rights and to fight for those who are unaware about their basic human rights.

No to Corruption

Although we all are facing some arduous times, it is very important to stay strong to endure this pandemic. We have to empathize that we share with each other the bond of humanity. It is the right time for the privileged class of the society to come forward and outreach the backward strata of the nation which are suffering the most. If wealthy people contribute more then this will lead to pool of financial sources and thus in turn will help to prevent corruption at various levels.

10 | REMDESIVIR: "REMEDY FOR THE SEVERE"?

The novel coronavirus SARS-CoV-2 which has been originated from bats (Rhinolophus Affinis) in the Wuhan, Hubei Province of China in December 2019. Given it's aerosol mode of transmission (which later became completely air-borne), it spread to the entire globe and it was officially declared a pandemic by the World Health Organization on 11th March 2020. The sudden eruption of such global disaster created worldwide agitation. As there was no anticipation of such a global emergency; the emergence of COVID-19 created a ruckus especially in the health-care sector. Lack of exclusive research led to unavailability of sufficient literature pertaining to the novel corona virus.

Coronavirus belongs to the family "Coronaviridae" and genus "Betacoronavirus" which consists of a group of enveloped viruses with a positive sense, single stranded RNA genome which can affect animals as well as human beings. The other members of the Coronaviridae family includes virus responsible for common cold, severe acute respiratory syndrome coronavirus (SARS CoV), Middle East respiratory-syndrome related coronavirus (MERS CoV) and the latest Severe acute respiratory syndrome coronavirus 2 (SARS-CoV-2) which is the causative pathogen for COVID-19. The SARS-CoV-2 has **79.6%** similarity with SARS CoV virus.

Remdesivir(GS-5734) is a prodrug which was patented by the Gilead Sciences Inc., US in collaboration with U.S. Centers for Disease Control and Prevention (CDC) and the U.S. Army Medical Research Institute of Infectious Diseases (USAMRIID). It is an investigational nucleoside analogue which is a drug that inhibits reverse transcription thus inhibiting the virus. Its development was done while combating the spread of Ebola virus.

What are "in vitro" & "in vivo" studies?

Before moving on to the actual working and potency of Remdesivir, we have to understand what are the different types of investigative studies done to decide whether a particular drug is effective for treating a particular disease or infection.

The efficacy of remdesivir has been proven both in vitro as well as in vivo studies. As far as in vitro studies are concerned, the use of remdesivir has shown positive effects in terms of both prevention as well as treatment. It has shown promising results in curbing the growth of SARS-CoV virus by inhibiting RNA replication. But as far as experimentation of remdesivir on human subjects is concerned; the available data of clinical and control trials is inadequate to establish the potency of the drug. WHO have not recommended the use of remdesivir for treating COVID-19 patients due to lack of sufficient clinical data. But the U.S. Food and Drug Administration (FDA) gave a green flag for the use of remdesivir as an "emergency medicine" for mild cases of COVID-19.

Mechanism of Action of Remdesivir

The WHO had conducted various "Solidarity" clinical trial studies to find out the efficacy of various drugs including Remdesivir in treatment of COVID-19. Remdesivir is a prodrug, i.e. it can't have any chemical effect in its original form. In order to remdesivir to act against the COVID-19 virus, it has to undergo change under the influence of certain enzymes. These enzymes are present in the human body. Once remdesivir is administered by intra venous mode, it is acted upon first by esterase followed by kinase and converted to its active form which is known as "**GS-441524**".

On the other hand, COVID-19 virus which has already been internalized by the human body, releases viral RNA. The transcription of this viral RNA is facilitated by the enzyme "**Viral RNA-dependent RNA polymerase (RdRp)**". Active form of remdesivir i.e.GS-441524 binds with RdRp by binding with it. As the influencer enzyme (RdRp) is translated into inactive form, there is no further replication of viral RNA and this leads to premature termination of RNA replication. Furthermore, the GS-441524 gets incorporated into the RNA strand. And this leads to neutralization of the COVID-19 virus.

Is Getting Remdesivir So Important?

Although remdesivir is known to have shown some positive effects in vitro; there is no report of any clinical trial in vivo which has supported the claim that remdesivir can prove life-saving in severe cases of COVID-19. The absence of a concrete prophylactic or curative alternative for treating COVID-19 seems to somehow convince people that remdesivir is the only way out for a patient with COVID-19 infection. It should be made very clear that remdesivir is effective in terms of reducing the recovery time only in mild cases of the disease. i.e. If a patient is given remdesivir within first ten days of the disease then his condition is seen to improve after 10 days whereas another patient who is not given remdesivir takes 15 days. It is also not proven that remdesivir has any role in severe cases of COVID-19. So, before falling prey to false claims and before developing the guilt of not being able to arrange remdesivir for any critical COVID-19 patient we have to keep in mind that-

1. U.S. Food and Drug Administration (FDA) has approved the "**emergency use**" of remdesivir for treating COVID-19 cases in spite of inadequacy of clinical trial data on the efficacy and potency of the same.

2. World Health Organization (WHO) has not recommended the use of remdesivir in severe cases of COVID-19 given the fact that it has got no effect on curbing the advanced symptoms in terminally ill patients.

3. Remdesivir is known to reduce the recovery time in mild to moderate cases of COVID-19.

4. Remdesivir is only effective if given within the first 10 days of the infection.

5. Remdesivir has got both prophylactic as well as curative effect in vitro whereas it has shown only curative effect in vivo (only in mild cases that too if administered within first 10 days since the development of symptoms).

6. Thus, considering the factors mentioned above, the claim of remdesivir being the ultimate life-saving drug in cases of COVID-19 patients is a hoax and completely baseless.

7. These scientific facts need to be circulated in the public as much as possible in order to curtail black marketing and money-minting business going on nowadays in the society.

8. Also it will help to relieve the guilt off individuals who have lost their family member because of their failure to arrange a vial of remdesivir for treatment.

11 | COVISHIELD, COVAXIN OR 'NO' VACCINE?

Why to get Vaccinated? – The Million Dollar Question

Healthcare system is on the verge of collapse as India is witnessing the second wave of the COVID-19 pandemic. As of 10th May 2021, India ranks second in the list of most number of COVID-19 cases with USA topping the chart. As per the data provided by the National Informatics Centre (Ministry of Electronics & Information Technology, Government of India), approximately 17 crore people in India have been vaccinated till 10th May,2021 which comprise about 12.5% of the total population of India. This huge gap between the actual demand of vaccine and production needs to be narrowed. Although the scarcity of vaccine won't offer the option of choice to the people, it is still important to know about the various options available in the market in order to clear the dilemma related to vaccine.

Currently various companies like Bharat Biotech and Serum Institute of India are the leading vaccine manufacturers and suppliers in India. The various vaccine brands like Covishield (Serum Institute of India), Covaxin (Bharat Biotech) and Sputnik V (developed by Gamaleya Research Institute of Epidemiology and Microbiology, Russia) are being administered to the Indian population.

It is a general belief that getting vaccinated makes you fully immune to that particular disease. But, there have been quite a few cases wherein individuals have been tested positive in spite of having completed the vaccination schedule. So several questions need to be answered such as which vaccine brand to prefer? How much gap should be kept between the two doses? or the rudimentary question – whether to get vaccinated or not?

Why to get Vaccinated?

Looking at the current rate of spread of COVID-19, experts have predicted that it is most likely that India might experience the third wave by the beginning of November or late December 2021. Contrary to the condition prevailing in rest of India, the capital Delhi has already witnessed fourth wave of COVID-19. Shortage of beds, ventilators and oxygen as well as black marketing of Remdesivir, Tocalizumabetc are making the conditions worse in India's capital city. As various measures to control the exponential spread of the virus have been failed so far, researchers have predicted that achieving herd immunity is the only viable option right now to stop the COVID-19 pandemic. The following factors will help to clear the doubts related to vaccination against COVID-19.

1. *Herd Immunity*

"Herd immunity" which is also known as "population immunity" is a type of mass immunity developed by a specific percentage of the population either because of vaccination or due to developing immunity following the contraction of the disease, so that the remaining percentage of population get automatically immune to the virus without vaccination or acquiring the disease. As far as COVID-19 is concerned, it is strongly recommended by the World Health Organization (WHO) that every country should strive to achieve herd immunity by maximizing their efforts for vaccinating the population. This is because if we wait for the development of active immunity it may further add up to the mortality rate.

Now, for herd immunity to work out; a significant threshold value is set for each disease depending upon the severity of the strain of the virus. e.g. for a population to acquire herd immunity against polio virus, it was necessary that at least 80% of the population develops immunity either through vaccination or by developing active immunity after getting the disease. The rest of the 20% population will be protected even if they don't develop active immunity or get vaccinated as the spread of virus will cease among the 80% immunized population.

This **herd immunity threshold** is difficult to calculate in case of coronavirus given it's various highly infective and constantly mutating strains. Attempts are constantly being made to obtain a definite herd immunity threshold for COVID-19. In 2020, the herd immunity threshold for COVID-19 was calculated to be 60–70% which has now increased to 80–90% in 2021. So, for now vaccination of the masses is the only choice to combat this devastating pandemic.

2. Alleviate Associated Complications

The second major advantage of getting vaccinated is the severity of associated complications during the COVID stage as well as post-COVID stage gets significantly reduced. Studies have shown that individuals who have been vaccinated showed higher recovery as compared to those who were not vaccinated. Prevalence of associated complications like breathlessness, pneumonia, development of clots, mucormycosis etc. reduces drastically in vaccinated individuals than non-vaccinated individuals.

3. Reduce Mortality

As the associated symptoms are alleviated, the mortality rate goes further down if the individual is vaccinated. Usually mortality in COVID-19 patients is due to aggravation of the symptoms. The ultimate course of the disease is ventilator support and multi-organ failure.

4. Safety of the Vulnerable Group

The main safety concern nowadays is of the highly vulnerable group of people with co morbidities as well as geriatric population. These are the groups which have the highest rate of mortality as the progression of the disease is rapid owing to the general debility and immunocompromised status secondary to prevailing co morbidities. Being vulnerable group, they also cannot be vaccinated as the dose itself may induce life-threatening side effects in them. This is the reason why the safety of this vulnerable group depends solely on the immunization of the rest of the population.

5. To Avoid being an "Unaware Super-spreader"

A responsible individual; who is well aware of his responsibilities towards the society, knows that each and every action of his ultimately affects the society. So, if you are having symptoms you need to isolate yourself from others. But what if the individual is asymptomatic? Even if he follows all the precautions when in public, he can still transfer the virus to his family while inside the house. This is where vaccination plays a very crucial role to prevent you from becoming an "**unaware super-spreader**".

6. To Avoid being a "COVIDIOT"

"Covidiots" are those who do not follow the safety guidelines as prescribed by the various health regulatory bodies and thus are responsible for the further spread of COVID-19. This is the final reason why we need to get vaccinated. We are facing some unusually tough times and we are in this together. So, we need to take collective responsibility of the society and contribute in breaking the chain by getting vaccinated.

12 | THE CHAIN THEORY

Sequentially Altered Biomechanics & Mechanical Low Back Pain during COVID-19 lockdown

Lockdown has caused a complete stoppage of our social lives. "Work from home" concept has been adopted by major multi-national corporate companies. As this new lifestyle has made us more sedentary, chances of development of musculoskeletal disorders has elevated significantly.

Low Back Pain (LBP) has been a major cause of debility in global population. Specifically, the mechanical variant is more prevalent in the society. Altered lifestyle, reduced physical fitness, obesity etc are the contributing factors for non-pathological LBP. While taking history of a patient of mechanical or non-specific low back pain; we tend to focus upon the recent traumatic history. When it comes to biomechanical aspect of various contributory factors for LBP, the sequence has to be considered and not just the recent history of pain.

It is hypothesized that for non-specific or mechanical low back pain to develop, either the Up-chain or the Down-chain phenomenon has to be the etiological factor. The chain of events (structural or biomechanical changes) can occur either in an ascending order or descending order over a period of time. It is not necessary that a person will check through all the symptoms throughout the course of biomechanical alterations. It is possible that an individual might skip a step or two and jump over the next effect. It can vary individually depending upon various factors.

A. Up-chain effect

B. Down-chain effect

The proposed theory states that "Any painful musculoskeletal or neurological condition pertaining to the central axis of the body i.e. vertebral column is a result of sequential, inter-dependent alterations that occur in terms of biomechanics of various structures over a period of time."

The Up Chain Effect

The Up chain effect; as the name suggests, refers to development of alterations in biomechanics of the various joints in a ascending order. i.e. from the lower side of the body first then progressing towards the upper side of the body.

1. Outward deviation of the foot from the saggital axis in the coronal plane.

2. Throughout the length support of the Hamstring

3. Abducted Hips

4. Reduced/Exaggerated Lumbar lordosis

5. Scapular Retraction

6. Position of Optimal Functioning (POOF) of the Pectoralis Major muscles.

The Down Chain Effect

The down chain effect refers to the gradual development of biomechanical alterations starting from the upper part of the body.

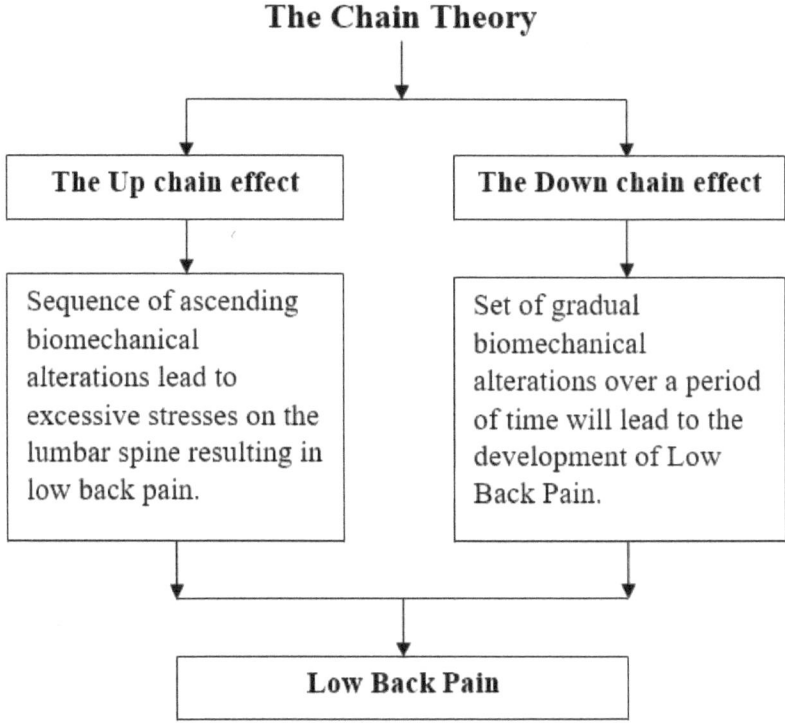

Flowchart 1.1. The Chain Theory

As mentioned earlier, both of these are hypothesis and need strong research support to be proven. But, it can be considered as an "early warning sign" so that efforts can be started for its prevention or treatment.

13 | THE DECONDITIONING FUNNEL EFFECT

It is usually thought that athletes are highly evolved human beings and are less prone to various illnesses and infections as compared to non-athletic population. Although it might hold true to some extent (as far as minor infections are concerned), the emergence of COVID-19 pandemic has totally shattered this myth of low-vulnerability of the athletes to various illness & infection. Entry of SARS-CoV-2 inside of a cell is facilitated by angiotensin converting enzyme-2 (ACE-2) receptor which majorly resides in the heart, endothelial cells and is responsible for inflammatory response activation.[1] Athletes are equally vulnerable for the subsequent complications of COVID-19; as other non-athletic population, which can trigger an exaggerated inflammatory response which could ultimately lead to myocardial infarction.[2]

Secondary to the forced lockdown imposed by the governments of various countries worldwide, deteriorating changes have been seen in athletes in terms of maximal oxygen consumption (VO_{2max}), endurance as well as muscle strength and mass.It is therefore a very alarming factor for the athletes to ponder upon in order to prevent further deterioration of their overall performance in their respective field of sports. Myocarditis is serious complication which might be the cause of sudden cardiac death in competitive athletes with a normal ventricular function.

Restricted space and unavailability of tools & resources are the two major obstacles which have been experienced by people willing to continue their pre-lockdown workout routine during the tough COVID times. World Health Organization (WHO) has published recommendations for daily physical activity by overcoming the above mentioned problems.To maintain a healthy routine, WHO recommends a 150-min of moderate intensity or 75-min of vigorous intensity physical activity (PA) during home isolation. Furthermore, to achieve additional health benefits; 300-min of moderate intensity or 150-min of vigorous intensity PA is recommended. A daily workout routine can be designed by taking into consideration the following factors:

1. Age of the individual

2. Availability of resources

3. Surrounding area of isolation

4. Presence of co-morbidity

5. Feasibility

6. Economic stability of the individual

The role of a Sports Physiotherapist is to ensure the maintenance of optimal performance parameters of an athlete by designing routine home-training protocol to circumvent "**the deconditioning-funnel effect**" which has been described in detail later. The concept of "**Non-Exercise Activity Thermogenesis (NEAT)**" can be utilized as a potent tool for designing moderate to high intensity PA protocols for both athletic as well as non-athletic population during home isolation.

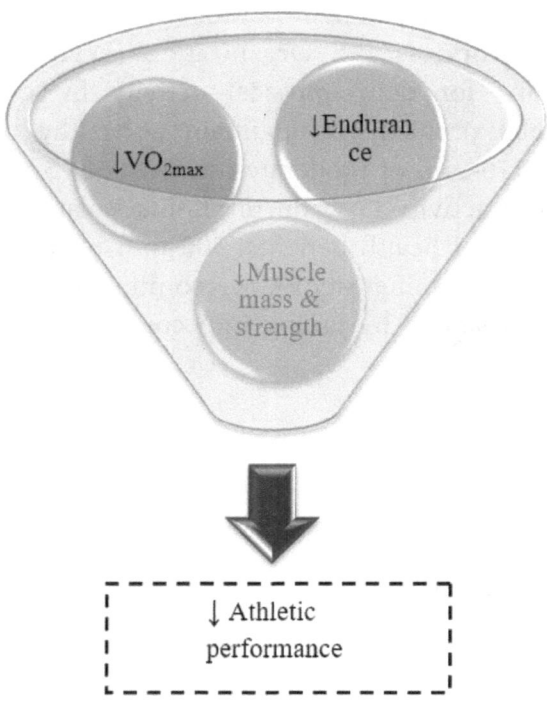

Figure.4.1 The Deconditioning-funnel effect

"The Deconditioning-funnel effect" is believed to be the primary reason behind the reduced performance of athletes during the lockdown period. It has been coined by Dr. PrasannajeetNikam (2020). $VO_{2max,}$ cardio-pulmonary endurance and muscular power and strength are the key parameters which determine the competitive performance of an athlete. Prolonged detraining which resulted due to imposition of lockdown led to a significant disruption of the physical as well as psychological abilities among the athletic population. Athletes belonging to middle class and/or lower class were affected more because of the lack or unavailability of training resources. Reduced maximum oxygen intake capacity or $VO_{2max,}$ cardiopulmonary endurance and muscle mass & strength conjugate resulting in decreased physical performance of an athlete. If we try to conserve all the three parameters, we could be able to avoid "the deconditioning-funnel effect."

14 | PSEUDO-COVID SYNDROME

A Hidden Disaster

Winston Churchill, the most succinct Prime Minister of Great Britain, wrote that "Now this is not the end. It is not even the beginning of the end. But it is, perhaps, the end of the beginning." The analogy of the above mentioned quote and today's prevalent circumstances is surreal. There comes a point where we see the mirage of COVID-19 cases being controlled, but suddenly this this bubble is burst by the existence of "**Persistent Post-COVID Syndrome**".

Oronsky et al (2021) has coined a new term called as "**persistent post-COVID syndrome (PPCS)**". Just like post-sepsis syndrome and post-ICU syndrome, significant deterioration in the quality of life (QOL) and increased risk of mortality due to development of a group of associated complications may persist in COVID-19 survivors long after the infection has been subsided. This constellation of effects which leads to a morbid course during the post-ICU phase in COVID-19 survivors has been given the umbrella terminology of "**persistent post-COVID syndrome (PPCS)**".

So, there is sufficient scientific literature to prove that COVID-19 can have some serious interlinked long term effects which might lead even to death if not given adequate medical attention in time.

But, the main drawback of the PPCS is it inclusive only of the systemic physical effects of long-COVID. The post-COVID phase is known to have detrimental effects on the physiological QOL as well. At times, the intensity of the psychological involvement might be to such an extent that it may be precipitated as physical symptoms.

In order to demarcate between genuine manifestations of the disease and perception of psychologically precipitated symptoms of COVID-19, a separate terminology called as "Pseudo-COVID Syndrome(**PCS**)". The syndrome consists of constellation of various symptoms like-

1. Sore throat or a constant itch feeling at the back side of your tongue.

2. Intermittent costo-chondral pain (triggered on deep inspiration)

3. Headaches (mostly cervicogenic)

4. Abrupt feeling of lethargy or Body pain

5. Sense of joint pain.

6. Bouts of dry cough.

Stress or coronaphobia might manifest as a precursor to the Pseudo-COVID Syndrome. PCS along with coronophobia, Post-COVID syndrome and Persistent Post-COVID syndrome can collectively prove to be the major mental health risk factors during this pandemic.

15 | THE BLIND SPOT EFFECT

Our focus on COVID-19 has diverted our minds from other associated complications of covid-19 like Mask Man Syndrome, Foggy-Glass Syndrome, and Pseudo-Hypoventilation Syndrome (PHS). We are so haunted by the fear of contracting COVID-19 virus that we have lost the judgment of extent to which one should practice precautionary measures against the disease. Good things are not always good. Anything done in excess has its own harms. The Blind Spot Effect can be described as the inability to perceive the other equally dangerous consequences, due to entire focus on a single entity. In order to get a clear idea

Over-protective Measures – Good or Bad?

COVID-19 has been prevailing for about a year now and people appear to be adjusting to the modified lifestyle. Although the level of awareness about self-hygiene has increased as compared to what it used to be prior to COVID-19 pandemic, still a lack of uniformity can be seen in the practice of precautionary measures. Frequent washing of hands, disinfection of surrounding, use of appropriate facial masks, maintenance of social distancing etc are the essential safety practices recommended by the World Health Organization (WHO). But the question which still remains unanswered is how to quantify the extent of precautionary measures?

Understanding the Other Side of the Coin

After a thorough literature search, it was found that there have been recommendations regarding safety measures to be taken to reduce the spread of COVID-19. But no guidelines have been found which have focused exclusively on the demarcation between obligatory and imperative practice of such measures. People should be made aware of the possible complications on the various systems of the body due to following over-precautionary measures against COVID-19. Awareness has to be spread about the manifestation of such initially less severe looking symptoms into potentially adverse complications over a period of time. Self-consciousness about the mask on-off duration, judicious use of hand-sanitizers, frequency of disinfection, work from home schedule etc need to be kept a track of.

Possible Ill-effects of Over-Precautionary Measures

We have to understand that each and everything has got its own limits. If we cross that line then we better be ready to face the consequences. As far as practice of safety or precautionary measures is concerned, it has to be demarcated as to what extent the precautionary measures should be adopted. Secondary deteriorating effects are emerging in people who follow obsessive compulsive behavior related to precautionary measures against COVID-19. A specific set of signs and symptoms have been identified in people who share a common cause of compulsive safety measures. These syndromes mainly affect the musculoskeletal system and respiratory system to some extent. Such emerging syndromes have been discussed in details in the upcoming chapters.

Constant keeping mask-on might lead to accumulation of the exhaled CO_2 inside the mask space. Individual might feel a feeling of breathlessness due to rising CO_2 levels in the body which gives rise to a phenomenon called as "**Pseudo-Hypoventilation Syndrome**". The details of this emerging terminology has been described further.

a. *Pseudo-Hypoventilation Syndrome (PHS)*

The term "Pseudo-Hypoventilation Syndrome" has been coined collectively for all the possible direct as well as indirect effects seen on the musculoskeletal as well as respiratory system of an individual secondary to wearing masks for a prolonged period of time. It can be possibly seen in individuals who wear masks for a significant part of the day. Although it might take months or years altogether to develop the signs and symptoms of the above said syndrome, it should be looked upon as a possible threat and prophylactic modifications should be initiated at the earliest. The reason behind referring to it as a "pseudo" phenomenon is that it occurs without any underlying pathology of the respiratory system. It is a temporary condition and symptoms may cease to stop once the causative factors are eliminated.

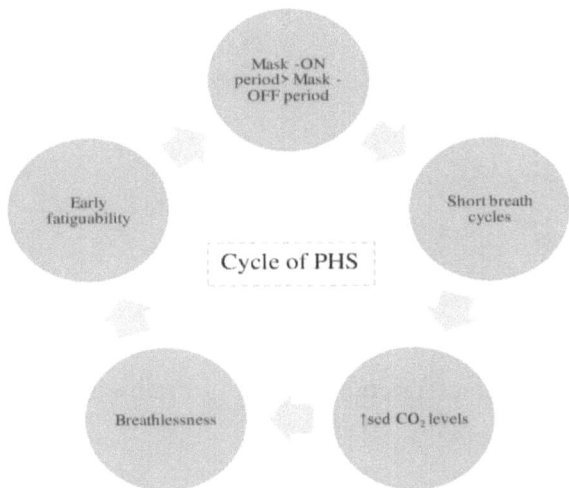

Theory of Etiology of Pseudo Hypoventilation Syndrome

(PHS)

The possible theory which is hypothesized for development of PHS is prolonged wearing of facial masks without intermittent mask-off period. The high risk population being the frontline healthcare professionals like Doctors, nurses, paramedics, janitors, sanitization department etc. The masks act like a closed environment trapping the exhaled CO_2, which in turn gets re-inhaled by the individual.

The mask-ON period is the duration for which an individual wears the facial mask whereas the mask-OFF period is the duration for which an individual doesn't wear the mask (takes off the mask). If the Mask-ON: Mask-OFF is ≥ 1 then the individual is vulnerable to develop the PHS. The ratio can be used as a screening tool to assess the potential risk of an individual for developing the various signs and symptoms of PHS.

The breath cycle i.e. inspiration and expiration time duration reduces as the body tries to compensate the dropping O_2 levels by increasing the respiratory rate. This is a mechanism triggered by the body to ensure optimal O_2 supply to the body.

The shallow breathing furthermore leads to increased CO_2 accumulation in the body. This leads to breathlessness secondary to hypoventilation causing early fatigability of the various muscles of the body.

Signs and Symptoms

1. Shallow-breathing or shortness of breath.

2. Tiredness

3. Mild feeling of heaviness of chest while attempting deep inspiration.

4. Chronic adverse effects may include reduced lung volumes and capacities.

DO's & DON'T's

1. Try to keep the Mask-ON: Mask-OFF ratio as low as possible by adding small bouts of deep inspiration and expiration breaks. These breaks have to be performed every 30 minutes throughout your daily schedule.

2. Practice deep inspiratory and forced expiratory exercises on a daily basis for 3–4 times a day.

3. Try to inculcate exercises which would mimic various physiological movements of the ribs like pump-handle and bucket handle movements.

b. Mask-Man Syndrome

Introduction

Novel Corona Virus pandemic has affected all strata's of life socially, economically as well as psychologically. The practice of sanitization, social distancing and optimal nutrition are the key habits which will ensure prevention of spread of this dreadful disease. Initially the mode of transmission of this disease was thought to be the aerosol effect through droplets which spread because of coughing or sneezing. The aerosol may remain viable in the open air for upto 3 hours. Later it was concluded that the novel virus is air-borne and can spread through normal breathing also. So the three hygienic steps of frequent hand-washing with sanitizer, maintenance of social distance and wearing of mask have been promoted and insisted by the governments of all countries in order to prevent the spread of this novel virus.

People belonging to the middle and lower-middle class as well as those from the below poverty line section of the society are facing additional challenges in coping up with this pandemic. Most people prefer homemade masks as they are less economically burdening. Being home-made, special consideration is not given on the features like fitting, comfort etc. This might lead to development of various face-mask related symptoms. The population who over-use facial masks are automatically at a higher risks of developing this cluster of inter-related signs and symptoms which has been termed as "Mask-Man Syndrome".

Mask-Man Syndrome

The lack of concrete information along with the absence of prophylactic drug has led to the spread of a wave of fear and misconceptions among the population throughout the world. As a result of this, the phenomenon of over-practice of hygienic habits or precautionary measures is been seen among the people. This includes continuous use of mask even in non-crowded or open areas like highways, gardens, farms etc; over utilization of hand-rubs or sanitizers etc.

The continuous wearing of masks like KN-95, N-95, cloth mask, surgical mask etc has its own disadvantages which haven't been studied till date. A list of signs and symptoms have been identified which are associated with over-use of mask. Various factors like duration of wearing face mask, type of mask, type of straps and fitting have an impact on the development of one or more of the following enlisted signs and symptoms.

Symptoms

1. Feeling of shortness of breath. (Pseudo-breathlessness)

2. Pain over the tip of the nose.

3. Retro-auricular or retro-pinnal pain.

4. Cervicogenic headache.

5. Neck pain.

6. Runny-nose after removal of mask following prolong use.

Any one or all of the above mentioned symptoms may co-exist in an individual. Symptom no.4 and 5 have been noted in people with powered eyewear or those who use sunglasses throughout the day. The area needs to be investigated by conducting surveys. It becomes necessary to identify the signs and symptoms by modifying the various causative factors. It can also be hypothesized that there could be possible deteriorating effect on the inspiratory or expiratory capacities of the lung.

Physiotherapeutic Approach

1. Contrast Bath, which is also known as "Hot/Cold Immersion method" can be used to reduce the strain on the primary pressure areas like the tip of the nose, pinna of the ear or any part of the face.

2. Basic self-massage techniques like effleurage can be prescribed after every 1–2 hours.

3. This will reduce the strain on the facial muscles as well as surrounding structures like the neck, ear etc.

Precautions to be taken

1. Usage of masks should be strictly limited to crowded places or closed spaces only.

2. Instead of preferring a specific type, different masks with varying structure should be used.

3. Prefer masks with open knots which need to be tied behind the head and not the one which come with a side loop to be worn around the ears.

4. A "Deep Breath Break" is advised especially for that working class of corporate population who are not accessible to "work from home" option and thus need to go to their respective workplaces.

5. Application of moisturizer over the pressure-prone areas might help to reduce the inconvenience secondary to prolong wearing of mask.

c. Foggy-glass Syndrome

Novel Corona virus Disease (COVID-19) has been prevailing in the society since a long time. It has exhibited the direct as well as indirect catastrophic effects it can possibly have on the human population. Researchers from all over the globe are constantly in a quest to obtain prophylactic as well as curative information regarding this novel virus. Hygienic practices like frequent hand-washing, social distancing and utilization of facial mask have been adapted as a part of routine throughout the world. Improved awareness about self-hygiene can be seen in various strata of the society.

As there are positive as well as negative aspects to everything, these adapted prophylactic measures may have adverse effects. This necessitates the conduction of prospective studies to figure out the possible associated adverse effects such adaptations might have on the health of the society. Identification of such associated risk factors might help to design prophylactic measures to prevent the occurrence of the same.

Foggy-Glass syndrome is a set of symptoms which has been identified as a potential associated risk factor of lifestyle modifications which have been adapted as a precautionary measure against COVID-19. It is exclusively seen in individuals with prescription eye-wear or spectacles. The phenomenon of "foggy-glasses" which is frequently experienced after wearing facial-mask leads to the development of involuntary coping mechanisms by the individual which might contribute to musculoskeletal as well as respiratory problems in future. Thus, it becomes necessary to identify such alarming symptom or group of symptoms so that its origin can be traced down in order to ensure proper treatment.

Etiology

Individuals who wear powered eye wares (spectacles) face this exclusive problem of foggy glasses after wearing masks. It results in accumulation of vapor on the inner glass surface of the spectacles which leads to blurring of vision. At times, if the quality of glass used in the eye wear is poor then the accumulated vapor may leave the surface smudged. This leads to unclear vision or eyesight. As a counter-measure, the individual tries to first control the rate of breathing by increasing the duration between inspiration or expiration. If the problem persists, then another coping mechanism which might be incorporated by the individual is **oral breathing**.

If the problem still persists then a typical cervical extension phenomenon is adapted by the individual. This is done to adjust the vision through the available clear spaces on the glass of the eyewear. At times, even slight protraction of the neck might be evident. This might cause straining of the fascia and may end up in **cervico-genic headache**. Prevalence of mechanical neck pain might increase in such population due to altered bio-mechanics. Even myo-fascial restrictions may be seen in such target population.

Health-care professionals who have to work in COVID-19 wards are at higher risk of developing this syndrome. It is therefore mandatory to address this potential cause of debility. Early incorporation of precautionary measures might help to reduce the symptoms and thus in turn improve the professional outcome.

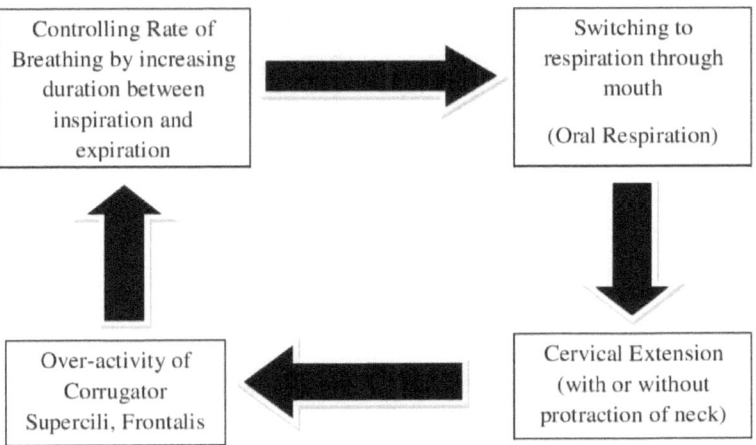

Cycle of etiology

Symptoms

 i. Shortness of Breath

 ii. Dryness of mouth

 iii. Mechanical neck pain

 iv. Cervicogenic headache

 v. Perception of tightness of chest while attempting deep inspiration.

Precautionary Measures

 i. Facial masks with nose-strip should be used as it will help to prevent the fogging in the first place.

 ii. Proper fitting masks should be used.

iii. Transcutaneous Electrical Nerve Stimulation (TENS) sessions can be given over neck region once a week as a prophylactic measure.

Role of Physiotherapy

i. **"Break the Streak"** regime should be advised where in prolonged, continuous hours of work should be broken down in relatively shorter durations with intermittent relaxation breaks. Breaks should include self stretching of the neck muscles like sternocleidomastoid, upper trapezius, corrugatorssupercili etc.

ii. Intermittent Forced Inspiratory bouts can be advised to maintain the basic vital lung volumes and capacities.

iii. Incentive Spirometry exercises should be performed on a daily basis in order to maintain vital capacities and volumes of lung.

iv. Self-massage for myo-fascial structures like frontalis, corrugator supercilietc can be advised.

v. Facial muscle exercises should be practiced.

Thus, owing to the possible complications it might impart on musculoskeletal as well as respiratory systems of an individual, "Foggy-Glass Syndrome" should be considered a potential barrier in deliverance of professional output especially in health-care providers. Apart from its therapeutic or rehabilitative role, Physiotherapy can play a prophylactic role in managing the various symptoms of "**Foggy-Glass Syndrome**".

16 | THE "DOT ON A BOARD" EFFECT

Time to Broaden the "Circle of Inclusion"

Imagine you are sitting in an empty classroom. There is a blackboard in front of you. Imagine a white dot at the centre of the board. When you keep staring at that particular dot for a prolonged duration, you notice that the dot appears to be expanding. At a point, you only see the dot and rest of the peripheral things become blurred. This is the "**dot on a board**" effect. There is an analogy between this effect and our current perspective on COVID-19. The way we are excessively focusing on COVID-19 has made us loose our peripheral vision which contain complications of COVID-19 like -

1. Myocardial Infarction (MI)

2. Stroke

3. Blood clots

4. Mucormycosis/Black fungus

5. Aspergillosis/White Fungus

6. MucorSepticus/Yellow fungus

7. Multi-organ failure

It is very crucial to anticipate the prevalence of these associated complications to help revive the patient before it's too late.

1. *Myocardial Infarction (MI)*

It is evident that viral pathogens like SARS may contribute to various cardiovascular conditions like acute myocarditis, acute myocardial infarction and rapid onset heart failure. COVID-19 is seen associated with cardiovascular events like myocardial injury, acute coronary syndromes, cardiac arrhythmias and heart failure. The possible explanation behind the development of cardiovascular complications in COVID-19 cases is expression of the ACE2 receptors which ultimately results in "**microvascular myocardial microcirculation disorder**" and other cardiac abnormalities.

2. *Stroke*

The neuro-invasive of the novel corona virus makes it easier to spread from the respiratory system to the neurovascular system and manifests in the form of febrile seizures, convulsions and encephalitis. Various series conducted in China and the US have described higher incidence of ischaemic or hemorrhagic stroke, Guillain-Barre syndrome (GBS) or acute necrotizing encephalopathy (ANE) in COVID-19 patients.

3. *Blood Clots*

Recent studies have erased the misconception of COVID-19 being purely a disease of the lungs. A report on COVID-19 autopsies showed that out of the total deaths, 58% individuals had deep vein thrombosis (DVT) which had further advanced to fatal venous thromboembolism (VTE) in 30% of the patients. Prophylactic Low Molecular Weight Heparin (LMWH) is known to be effective in preventing excessive clot formation as well as suppressing the inflammatory activity in the body.

4. *Mucormycosis*

"The Red Flag" of Black Fungus in COVID-19 patients

The black fungus disease is proving to be a separate pandemic on its own as the cases keep on rising on a daily basis. Symptoms include headache, fever, nausea, vomiting, swelling on one side of the face etc.

It is especially seen in case of people with co-morbidities and those who are immunocompromised.

5. White Fungus/Aspergillosis

White Fungus which is also called as "Aspergillosis" is believed to be way too dangerous than the black fungus but less severe complication than yellow fungus. Symptoms of white fungus include difficulty in swallowing, white patches on palate and/or tongue, sore throat fever etc.

6. Yellow fungus/MucorSepticus

Yellow fungus disease might initially manifest as unusual and easy fatigability, rashes, abnormal burning sensation on the skin etc. Prolonged use of steroids, contaminated environment, uncontrolled diabetes, dirty surroundings, unhygienic habits, imunnocompromised body and presence of comorboditiesmight be the causative factors for the development of yellow fungus disease.

7. Multi-organ Failure

The excessive production of early response proinflammatory cytokines (tumor necrosis factor [TNF], IL-6 and IL-1β) which is also called as **"cytokine storm"**. This ultimately results in increased risk of vascular hyper-permeability, multi-organ failure and death.

17 | THE "DIME A DOZEN" APPROACH TOWARDS MENTAL HEALTH AMIDST COVID-19 CHAOS

The outbreak of COVID-19 has flooded the entire ecosystem with various problems and challenges. The spectrum of these problems and challenges ranges from mild discomforts to severe life hindering complications. Since the declaration of the pandemic back in March 2020, people have been living under stressful circumstances for a better part of the year. COVID-19 has brought along with it massive psychological earthquake; remains of which will be prevailing for many decades.

COVID-19 has been rightly identified as a systemic disease which affects many systems of the body. This statement is contrary to the initial assumption of COVID-19 being a disease confining only to the respiratory system of an individual. The multi-system invasion of the novel coronavirus can be attributed to its affinity for the ACE 2 receptors (angiotensin converting enzyme 2) which is present in majority parts of a human body including most vital organs like brain and lungs. Even the ones without any genetic predisposing factor or the one who are psychologically robust have not been spared from developing psychological complications pertaining to COVID-19. At times it might be just another acute panic attack or it may be chronic infestation resulting in "**allostatic load**".

Another perplexity can be associated with the identification of stressors which induce any form of psychological agitation. It's generally a false notion which people tend to believe that there can be only genetic predisposing factors for development of any psychological issues in an individual. But, the arrival of COVID-19 has corroborated how scarcity of literature can help go any problem out of hand in no time. Anxiety, depression, post-traumatic stress and allostatic load are increasing in population due to various factors like virus infection, treatment with immune-suppressing drugs like corticosteroids, perception of uncertainty or loneliness in hospitals or isolation wards etc.

In order to know the severity of consequences inflicted by an unstable psychological status on human beings, it is very crucial to study how various systems of our body respond to different types of stressors. In case of threat or adverse circumstances, it is the neuroendocrine and immune system which responds primarily. The hypothalamic-pituitaryadrenal axis has a pathophysiologically crucial role in the development of allostatic load. Neurochemical functions of the brain are affected by both genomic as well as non-genomic mechanisms. Stress has deep effects in the long run which includes altered body functions pertaining to cardiovascular and gastrointestinal system. The endocrine metabolic balance gets disturbed thus ultimately affecting sleep patterns.

Coronaphobia

Coronaphobia can be defined as "irrational fear of acquiring the disease in spite of following all the necessary safety and precautionary measures." It takes a significant piece of mind of an individual, hindering his activities of daily living. It may lead to the development of Obsessive Compulsive Disorder (OCD) which may manifest as excessive practice of hygienic activities like frequent washing of hands, over use of sanitizers, constant fear, anxiety, etc.

COVID Stress Syndrome

COVID-19 has triggered a **"tsunami"** of psychological distress throughout the world. A study conducted in china showed that nearly 25% of the population were having moderate to severe stress- or anxiety-related symptoms secondary to COVID-19. A study by Taylor et al concluded that the COVID-19 stress syndrome is a complex phenomenon and cannot be limited to describing it as a simple one-dimensional fear of infection. It involves various types of fear, checking and reassurance seeking, and re-experiencing symptoms, along with other associated features such as excessive avoidance and panic buying.

Post-COVID Syndrome

It is evident that the total number of people affected psychologically can easily outnumber the total proportion of people infected with the disease. i.e. The psychological footprint of COVID-19 is much more than its physical footprint. Thus, it is very important to focus on the mental health aspect in each and every individual. It has been observed that the psychological health deterioration continues even after an individual recovers from COVID-19.

All of the conditions mentioned above are having serious mental impact on huge proportion of population and thus it has to be given equal importance that it deserves. Along with physical rehabilitation, it is also the psychological recovery that one should work on to strengthen during post COVID-19 rehabilitation phase.

18 | SMELL AND TASTE ACQUISITION THERAPY (STAT)

Gustatory & Olfactory Rehabilitation For COVID-19 Survivors

COVID-19 affects various systems of the body. The symptoms are inter-dependent. This is the reason why a multi-centric rehabilitation approach is advocated for COVID-19 patients. Studies have shown that the residual complications of COVID-19 may last up to 6 months to 2 years. This includes reduced lungs volumes and capacities, decreased muscular endurance, anxiety, depression etc. One of the main residual complications of COVID-19 is partial or complete loss of taste (**aguesia**) and smell (**anosmia**). The extent of inability to perceive taste and smell differs from person to person in case of COVID-19 infection. This therapy can be used both diagnostically as well as therapeutically.

Smell and Taste Acquisition Therapy (STAT)

Smell and Taste Acquisition Therapy (STAT) is an innovative home based rehabilitation approach designed to address the altered perception of smell and taste post COVID-19 infection. It includes re-training of the gustatory as well as the olfactory components by re-enforcing the smell and taste receptors of the body. It has two components-

A. **Olfactory rehabilitation component**

B. **Gustatory rehabilitation component**

Each of the two components has got three gradually progressing levels. They are-

Level 1 – Mild/Low

Level 2 – Moderate/Medium

Level 3 – Intense/Strong

Frequency/Dosage-It can be performed 3–4 times a day depending upon the severity of the condition.

Smell and Taste Acquisition Therapy (STAT)

A. *Olfactory Rehabilitation Component*

Level 1 – Mild/Low

    i. Flower (night lily or jasmine) – **1 point**

    ii. Coconut oil – **1 point**

    iii. Raw leafy vegetables like fenugreek, spinach – **1 point**

    iv. Butter/cheese – **1 point**

Level 2 – Moderate/Medium

    i. Curry leaves – **1 point**

    ii. Soap – **1 point**

    iii. Scented candles/incense sticks – **1 point**

    iv. Garlic/Ginger – **1 point**

Level 3 – Intense/Strong

    i. Eucalyptus leaves/Oil – **1 point**

    ii. Camphor – **1 point**

    iii. Coffee – **1 point**

    iv. Sanitizer – **1 point**

B. *Gustatory Rehabilitation Component*

Level 1 – Mild/Low

   i. Sugar – **1 point**

   ii. Fruits like banana or papaya. – **1 point**

   iii. Curds – **1 point**

   iv. Jams – **1 point**

Level 2 – Moderate/Medium

   i. Salt – **1 point**

   ii. Sauce – **1 point**

   iii. Fruits like pomegranate, mangoes – **1 point**

   iv. Buttermilk – **1 point**

Level 3 – Intense/Strong

   i. Lemon juice (without sugar) – **1 point**

   ii. Periperi or chaat masala – **1 point**

   iii. Soya/Chilli sauce – **1 point**

   iv. Bitter gourd – **1 point**

Procedure

- It is recommended that the patient should have a steam-inhalation prior to starting the STAT protocol. This will help to clear the oro-pharynx as well as the naso-pharynx and in turn increase the output of the therapy.

- Once the patient has taken the steam-inhalation or steam bath, he should wait for 5–10 min and then start with the first component i.e. olfactory rehabilitation component of the STAT protocol.

- The patient has to begin with level 1 i.e. mild/low. In this the patient has to tie a blind on his eyes such that he is not able to see. The other person has to ensure that there is no scope for cheating. This step is necessary to eliminate the factor of error.

- Once the patient has been blinded properly, then the person has to chose any random substance/thing from among the list and take it near the nose of the patient. The patient is not actively allowed to touch the substance/thing as he may perceive the thing through touch and might lead to faulty interpretations.

- Once taken near the nose of the patient, the other person has to ask the patient to gradually take a deep breath as if he is trying to smell the thing.

- If the patient is unable to identify or perceive the smell then he is given 3–4 more attempts. Each patient can be given a maximum of 5 attempts.

- Once the patient perceives the thing or if his 5 attempts get over then the other person has to move on to the next thing in the list and similar procedure has to be repeated.

- A gap of 5 min can be kept within the component. i.e. once done with the level 1, a person can wait for 5 min before progressing to level 2.

- A gap of 15 min is recommended between the components. i.e. once done with the gustatory component, a person has to wait or take a break of 15 min before starting the olfactory component.

- The STAT protocol can be performed 3–5 times a day depending upon the existing severity of the residual COVID-19 complications.

Scoring

- Each level has a maximum score of **4**.

- Each component has a maximum score of **12**.

- Maximum total score of STAT protocol is **24**.

Interpretation of Score

In STAT protocol, the individual level scores are more significant in determining the status of disorder than the total score. e.g. a total score of 16/24 won't give us any idea on the current status of taste and smell sense of the patient. However, a low score of level 1 or level 2 would indicate that the patient has still got high threshold for taste or smell as he is able to smell or taste only the strong/intense ones.

The only limitation of STAT protocol is it requires one more helping individual besides the patient. But it is practically non-existent as people are at their respective houses as a result of lockdown imposed throughout the globe. So, each patient can find an assistant in order to carry out this protocol. Rest assured, this protocol can help patients cope up with residual COVID-19 complications using the resources which are easily available at their respective homes.

Thus, Smell and Test Acquisition Therapy (STAT) can be incorporated as a routine workout to correct any altered sensations of taste and/or smell during the post COVID-19 rehabilitation phase.

19 | SUPPORTIVE-THERAPIES IN COVID-19

a. BREATHE – Supplementary Therapy for Reducing Psychological Stresses due to Corona Phobia

INTRODUCTION

COVID-19 cases have been increasing exponentially since the onset of this global pandemic. The healthcare workers have been working tirelessly in managing and rehabilitating COVID-19 positive patients. Although there has been an increase in the level of awareness among the population throughout the world, a mild apprehension is seen especially among the healthcare workers and medical service providers who work in close proximity of such patients for a prolonged period of time. This irrational fear of contracting the disease in spite of taking the appropriate precautionary safety measures has been termed as "Corona phobia".

Corona phobia has been known to possess a major psychological threat in recent times. It is mandatory to take necessary steps in order to reduce the possible psychological damage inflicted by corona phobia.

The following **BREATHE** checklist has been formulated by taking into consideration various factors which can directly or indirectly contribute towards the psychological well being of an individual. The components of the checklist are as follows:

B – Blind-eye towards social media

Social-media has its own pros and cons. At times it may provide beneficial and authentic information to the mass and help to prevent a certain catastrophe. On the other hand, misleading and fake information may add on to the already existing instability in the society. People have to become more aware and cautious in order to prevent worsening of the situation by believing hoax. The authenticity of particular information has to be seen before believing it or even forwarding it. Scientific literature with appropriate evidence should only be trusted before decision making.

R – Respiration

Forced inspiratory as well as expiratory capacities of the lung need to be improved. This can be achieved by practicing deep breathing exercises, yogasana etc. Breathing exercises help to increase the oxygen-retention levels and thus create a feeling of euphoria.

E – Eating

Diet should be holistic and balanced. This can be achieved by formulating a time table for the entire week wherein equal weightage should be given to fruits, fibers, proteins as well as minerals and vitamins. Try to keep the source as natural as possible. Avoid oily and junk food.

A – Attitude

The term "attitude" here refers to the mindset or the thought process which a person has to inculcate within. It basically refers to generating a concrete feeling of well-being and believing in it. If you are following the basic safety guidelines as advised by the World Health Organization (WHO) then there is no reason to pet irrational fear.

T – Training

Adequate aerobic conditioning of the body is very crucial as it proves to be a shield against the prevailing COVID-19 pandemic. As the primary system targeted by corona virus being the respiratory system, it is advised to keep the endurance boosted by practicing brisk walking or jogging for 30–45 minutes every day. Such long duration aerobic activity will help to improve the various volumes and capacities of the lung.

H – Habits

Habits refer to inculcating certain actions in day to day routine. It includes frequent washing of hands, wearing proper face-masks, social-distancing, multi-minerals and multi-vitamins intake, avoid addictions etc. But while following such hygienic activities a demarcating line has to be identified to prevent the possible complications of over-precaution against COVID-19. Prophylactic consumption of tablets like hydroxychloroquine, arsenic supplements etc should be avoided as it may affect the kidneys.

E – Emotional Hygiene

As people are becoming more concerned towards maintaining personal hygiene, emotional hygiene is not focused upon. Emotional hygiene refers to inculcating positive thoughts and a sense of psychological well-being. It is only when both, the mind as well as the body are disease-free that an individual is in harmony. Various interventions like relaxation techniques, Mental Imagery techniques, Virtual Reality devices etc can be used to sooth the mind and thus ultimately reduce stress and anxiety.

The above mentioned **BREATHE** checklist ensures a holistic approach towards combating the psychological complication of COVID-19 disease i.e. corona phobia. Although it has wide-spectrum applicability, it is especially beneficial for health-care providers who are the front-line warriors in this battle against COVID-19.

b. PhysiYoga: Shield against COVID-19 for the high-Risk Population

Introduction

Covid-19 still continues to be the primary agenda to address for all the countries throughout the world. The unavailability of sufficient concrete data regarding prophylactic as well as curative interventions for SARS-CoV-2 and COVID-19 disease has necessitated the exploration of alternative therapeutic options through conduction of research activities on a large scale.[1-4] Number of researchers are coming up with various strategies to combat the spread of this dreadful pandemic. Studies from China, Europe and the USA have established a consistently higher vulnerability of acquiring the COVID-19 infection in older individuals and those having underlying health conditions.[5-7] The various underlying co morbidities which increase the vulnerability of an individual to acquire COVID-19 disease are cardiovascular disease, chronic kidney, respiratory and liver diseases, cancer, HIV, tuberculosis, chronic neurological disorders and sickle cell disorders.[8] The high rate of mortality of COVID-19 cases can be attributed to a large number of population belonging to this category getting infected. A study was conducted to find out the global, regional and national estimates of population at increased risk of severe COVID-19 infection due to underlying health conditions.[9] It concluded that about one out of every five individuals has an underlying condition which could eventually put them at a higher risk of acquiring COVID-19 disease. The vulnerability was estimated to be less than 5% for individuals less than 20 years of age where as it was as high as 66% for older individuals having age 70 years and above. Thus, in order to control the mortality rate it becomes crucial to plan preventive self-help strategies in the form of a structured-routine which should be adopted by this high-risk population.

Many researchers have been focusing on the psychological effects of COVID-19 on general population as well as health-care professionals. Previous research studies which were carried out to see the psychological reactions to various epidemic and pandemic concluded that various psychological vulnerability factors may play a role in the development of coronaphobiaincluding individual difference variables such as intolerance of uncertainty, perceived vulnerability to disease and anxiety (worry) proneness.[10] Various psychosocial factors like disease associated stigmatization by the society may simply add up to the pre-existing anxiety, irritability and excessive feeling of stress or anger in the old age individuals. Lockdown effect has led to a wave of economic-crisis which has ultimately led to unemployment on a large scale. Restrictions imposed have led to decreased social life. All these factors may collectively have serious damage both physically as well as psychologically.

Indoor physical activity in the form of exercises might prove beneficial not only in maintaining the physical strength but also by alleviating the various psychological stresses especially in the older population.[11,12] Special emphasis need to be given on designing preventive as well as curative strategies which would target physical, psychological as well as psychosocial effects of COVID-19 in high risk population like quarantined people, health care professionals, children, older adults, marginalized communities and patients with previous psychiatric morbidities.[13]

This necessitated the development of a novel home-exercise approach incorporating physiotherapy as well as yoga in order to combat physical as well as psychological traits of human well-being. The integrated approach has been named as "PhysiYoga" and has been conceptualized and formulated by Dr.PrasannajeetPramodNikam.

PhysiYoga- Daily Routine Self-Care Protocol as a Shield against COVID-19 for the high-risk Population

PhysiYogais a novel daily routine self-care protocol which has been formulated by integrating physiotherapy and yoga with the ultimate aim of fortifying the individual physically, psychologically as well as psycho-socially. It is combination of activities intended to improve strength, balance, endurance, co-ordination, respiratory capacity as well as to generate a feeling of psychological well-being. The idea was to use physiotherapy for strengthening various systems and combine yoga to provide the psychological intervention divided over a period of one week. It consists of a group of strengthening, endurance, respiratory, balance and psychological exercises which any individual can perform by staying indoor. The yoga techniques included in this protocol are various types of breathing methods.

Components of PhysiYogaProtocol

Day	Physiotherapy Technique	Yoga Technique
Monday	1. Standing Wall Pushups 2. Biceps curls using Half-litre filled water-bottle 3. Incentive Spirometry – 3 sets*10 reps each	NadiSodhana Pranayama (20–30 repititions)
Tuesday	1. Brisk walking for 10 min 2. Wall support mini squats – 20 reps 3. Burpees – 3 sets*5 reps each 4. Incentive Spirometry – 3 sets*10 reps each	Ujjayi Pranayama (20–30 repititions)
Wednesday	1. Plank on bed – (30 sec–60 sec hold duration) 2. Cat-Camel exercises with alternate hand reachout (wearing half kg hand weight cuff) 3. Incentive Spirometry – 3 sets*10 reps each	Kapalabhati Pranayama (20–30 repititions)
Thursday	1. Twist and Raise walking technique – (30 reps) 2. Incentive Spirometry – 3 sets*10 reps each	Bhramari Pranayama (20–30 repititions)

Day	Physiotherapy Technique	Yoga Technique
Friday	1. Sit to Stand – 30–50 reps 2. Straight Leg Raises with ankle weight cuff (half Kg) – 30–50 reps 3. Incentive Spirometry – 3 sets*10 reps each	Sheetli Pranayama (20–30 repititions)
Saturday	1. Pelvic Bridging – 3 sets*10 reps each 2. Mckenzie Extension Regimen (3–5 reps) 3. Incentive Spirometry – 3 sets*10 reps each	Bhastrika Pranayama (20–30 repititions)
Sunday	1. Stepping – 30–50 reps 2. Tandem Walking 3. Incentive Spirometry – 3 sets*10 reps each	Dirga Pranayama (20–30 repititions)

Note:- Progression can be made as per suggestions of the consulting physiotherapist.

Benefits

This protocol encompasses various modes of training and thus will help to ensure to maintain optimum physical as well as psychological health status of the individual. The mode of delivery could be through video-calls or through short-videos explaining the guidelines about how to perform the exercises. This interaction between the patient and the therapist will help to reduce the psycho-social problems. Quest for holistic approach which includes involvement of various aspects of alternative medicines led to the formulation of this unique protocol. The physiotherapy exercises involved range from normal breathing exercises to low-intensity resistance training. The equipments used like water-bottle, pillow etc. can be found easily in the house thus making this protocol economically feasible.

20 | "LUNG-GYM" FOR COVID-19 SURVIVORS

Do It Yourself (DIY) Progressive Resistance Lung Exerciser
"HOME GYM" for your Lungs

Novel coronavirus, the severe acute respiratory syndrome coronavirus 2 (SARS-CoV-2), causing the Coronavirus Disease 2019 (COVID-19), has emerged in late 2019, which has posed a global health threat with its ongoing pandemic in many countries and territories. The symptoms include headache, fever, fatigue which may advance to severe complications like Acute Respiratory Distress Syndrome (ARDS) and even death. The chances of mortality get elevated if the person is having other co morbidities like diabetes, hypertension, Asthma etc.

The respiratory system is the one which gets infected primarily in this disease.

As there is no prophylactic or curative medicine available to combat this deadly disease, symptomatic treatment still remains the first line of management of this pandemic crisis.

Physiotherapy plays a very crucial role in the rehabilitation of COVID-19 patients.

As a rehabilitative intervention for improving the deteriorated respiratory capacity of the ICU patients, Incentive Spirometry is used.

The proposed invention titled **"Three Tier Covid-19 Progressive Resistance Lung Exerciser"** is conceptualized and designed with the aim of providing a economically feasible, multi-functional and sterile device which could provide resistance exercises to the lungs.

The device consists of materials which are easily accessible and readily available, cost-effective and re-usable. The proposed device can be used to give resisted exercises to the lungs thus increasing inspiratory as well as expiratory capacities.

TECHNICAL PROBLEM ADDRESSED

1. Pulmonary as well as respiratory rehabilitation determines the quality of recovery of the patient in ICU. Physiotherapist play major role right from initiating early ambulation in severe cases to clearing air-way in severe cases.

2. **COVID-19** patients , especially the one belonging to the lower-class or those who are below poverty line remain undervalued because financial constraints.

What choices do we have available in the market?

1. The first choice of modality used to train the pulmonary as well as respiratory parameters in ICU patients is the Incentive Spirometry.

2. Apart from this, various breathing exercises like Diaphragmatic breathing, Glossopharyngeal breathing etc are taught to the patients.

3. Blowing the balloon exercise is prescribed to the patients.

WHAT ARE THE DRAWBACKS/LIMITATIONS OF THESE KNOWN WAYS FOR SOLVING THE PROBLEM?

1. The Incentive Spirometer, on an average, costs about 450 rs to 1000 rs. It is not economically feasible especially to people who come from lower middle to lower class strata of the society.

2. Once the patient is moved out of the ICU then he/she is advised more complex set of exercises like functional training, endurance training etc thus limiting the use of incentive spirometer to the ICU only.

3. Incentive Spirometry can be used to improve the Forced Inspiratory Capacity of the individual. The major concern in COVID-19 patients is the lung elasticity or recoiling. And to address the same forced expiratory training needs to be provided which can't be administered using incentive spirometry.

4. Varying degree of resistance cannot be applied with the existing incentive spirometer.

5. Considering the rapidly increasing number of people getting infected with COVID-19, community-based rehabilitation is the urgent need and may become an integral part of rehabilitative aspect.

"HOME GYM" for your Lungs

The proposed "**THREE TIER COVID-19 PROGRESSIVE RESISTANCE LUNG EXERCISER**" is a simple, cost-effective device which can substitute the "Incentive Spirometer" as a relatively economically feasible, more safer (from contamination point of view) and dynamic equipment. The invention can prove very useful especially at the community-based rehabilitation in both urban as well as rural areas.

Components of each single unit consists of -

1. A body (plastic water bottle) filled with either cotton, water or semolina (rawa/sooji).

2. A mouth-piece (straw) to inhale or exhale air.

3. A rubber balloon tied at the other end of the mouth-piece (preferably straw) with the help of rubber.

The invention consists of three levels of resistance trainer units as follows-

1. Low Resistance

2. Moderate Resistance

3. High Resistance

All the components enlisted above are common for all the three units except the material with which the body is filled that changes. e.g. For low resistance unit, the material used to fill the body will be cotton, for moderate resistance water and for high resistance fine sand.

MECHANISM OF ACTION

The patient has to hold the first unit of the proposed device in hand. He/she has to forcefully blow out air by keeping the mouth-piece (straw) pursed in between the lips. When the patient does this, the forcefully exhaled air will travel from the mouth piece into the rubber balloon placed inside the body (plastic water bottle) surrounded by either cotton, water or fine sand. This will in turn inflate the rubber balloon. Once the patient has reached the end of his/her forceful expiratory phase, he/she has to inhale the same air without removing the mouth-piece. During the inspiratory phase, the recoiling of the rubber balloon along with the surrounding material will provide assistance to inspiring.

WHAT ARE THE NOVEL FEATURES OF THIS DEVICE?

1. The equipment is constructed with such materials which are easily available and readily accessible.

2. Unlike incentive spirometer which is used to train only the inspiratory capacity of an individual, the COVID-19 Lung Exerciser provides expiratory resistance training as well as inspiratory facilitation training.

3. As compared to the conventional incentive spirometer, this device is comparatively more safer to use and has less chances of spreading the infection as each and every component of it can be replaced after every single use.

4. As far as the conventional incentive spirometer is considered, it can provide exercises to improve inspiratory capacity alone. This proposed invention is unique as it provides resisted training to expiration as well as assists inspiration.

THREE TIER COVID-19 PROGRESSIVE RESISTANCE LUNG EXERCISER

BACKGROUND OF INVENTION

Novel coronavirus, the severe acute respiratory syndrome coronavirus 2 (SARS-CoV-2), causing the Coronavirus Disease 2019 (COVID-19), has emerged in late 2019, which has posed a global health threat with its ongoing pandemic in many countries and territories.[1]

The symptoms include headache, fever, fatigue which may advance to severe complications like Acute Respiratory Distress Syndrome (ARDS) and even death.

The chances of mortality get elevated if the person is having other co morbidities like diabetes, hypertension, Asthma etc.

The respiratory system is the one which gets infected primarily in this disease.

As there is no prophylactic or curative medicine available to combat this deadly disease, symptomatic treatment still remains the first line of management of this pandemic crisis.

Physiotherapy plays a very crucial role in the rehabilitation of COVID-19 patients.

As a rehabilitative intervention for improving the deteriorated respiratory capacity of the ICU patients, Incentive Spirometry is used.

The proposed invention titled "**Three Tier Covid-19 Progressive Resistance Lung Exerciser**" is conceptualized and designed with the aim of providing a economically feasible, multi-functional and sterile device which could provide resistance exercises to the lungs.

The device consists of materials which are easily accessible and readily available, cost-effective and re-usable.

The proposed device can be used to give resisted exercises to the lungs thus increasing inspiratory as well as expiratory capacities.

CLAIMS

1. Beneficial for ensuring outreach of physiotherapy rehabilitation at the community level.

2. Zero chances of spread of infection or contamination even to the same patient.

3. Feasible.

4. Easy to operate. No special training or manual required.

5. Non-invasive.

6. No side effects.

OBJECTIVE OF THE DEVICE

1. To providea economically feasible, multi-functional and sterile device which could provide resistance exercises to the lungs.

2. To ensure the outreach of low cost physiotherapy intervention at the community level.

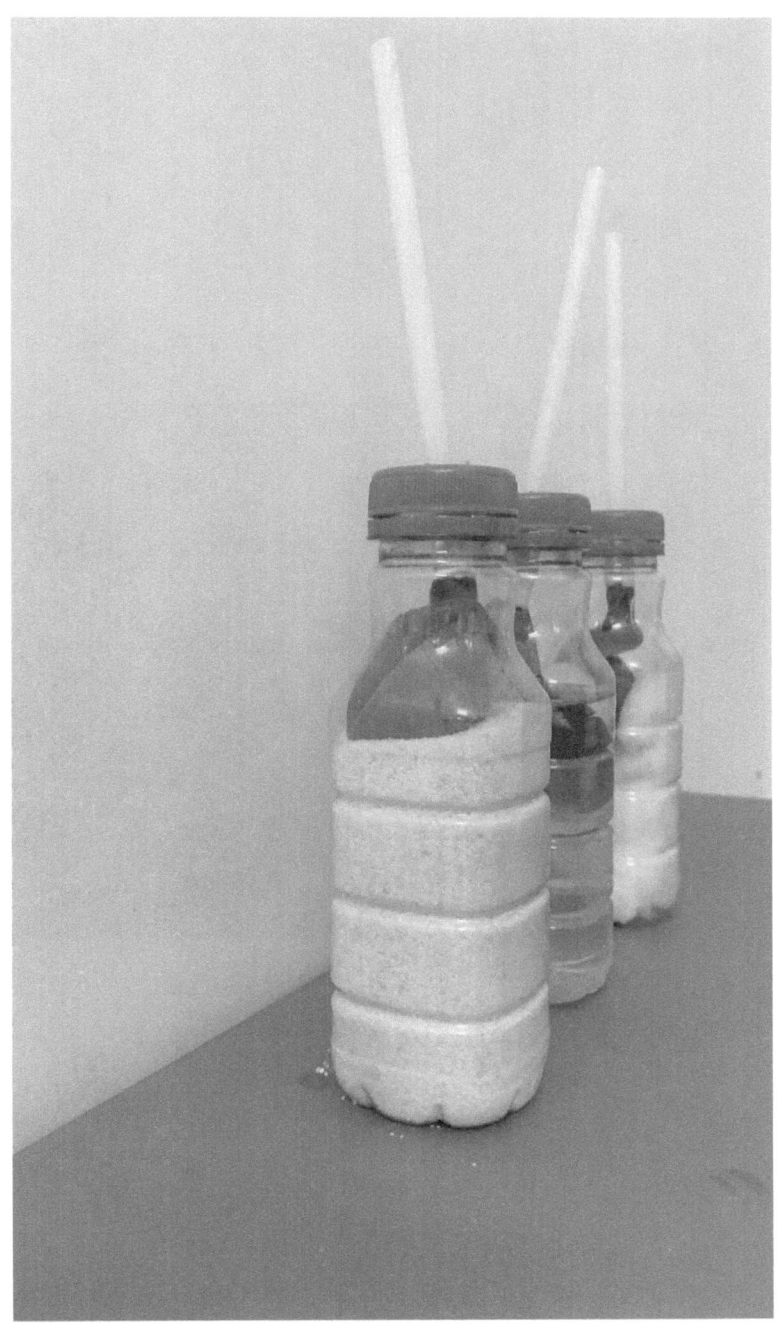

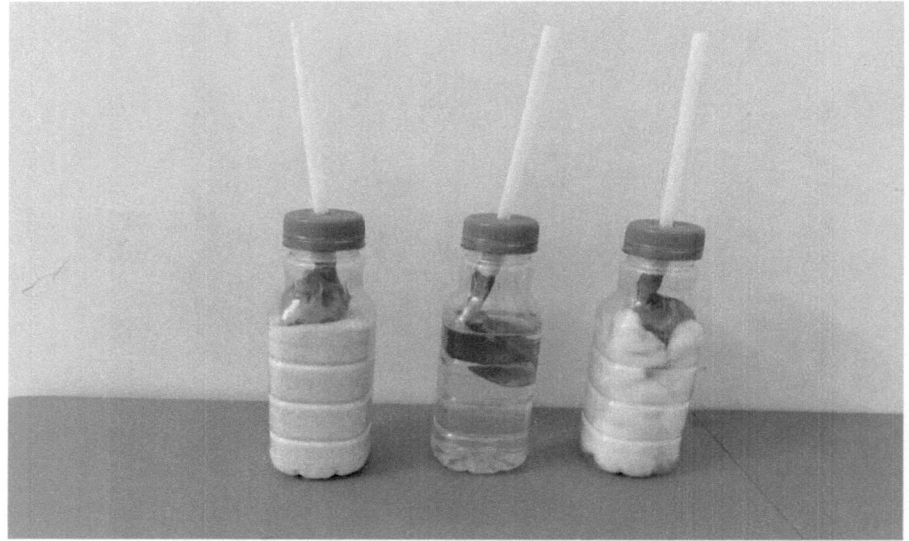

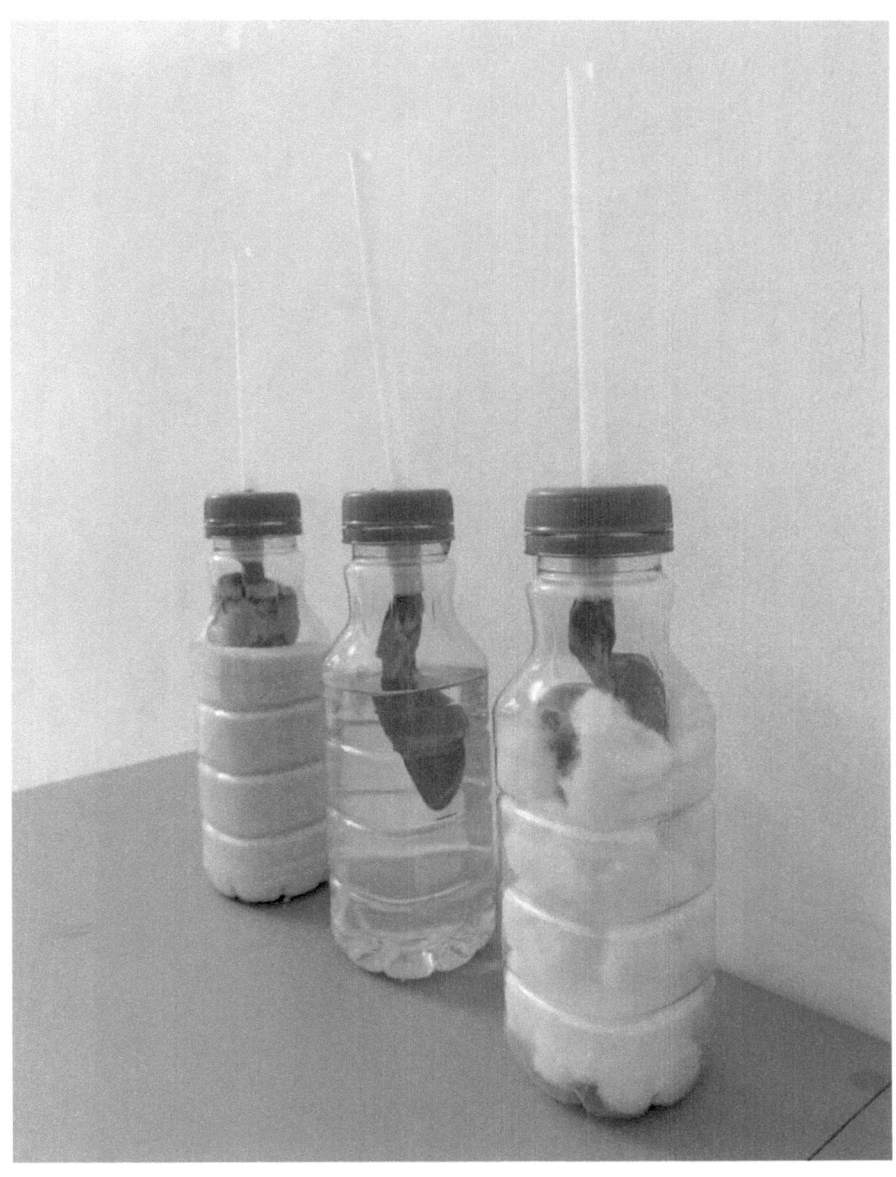

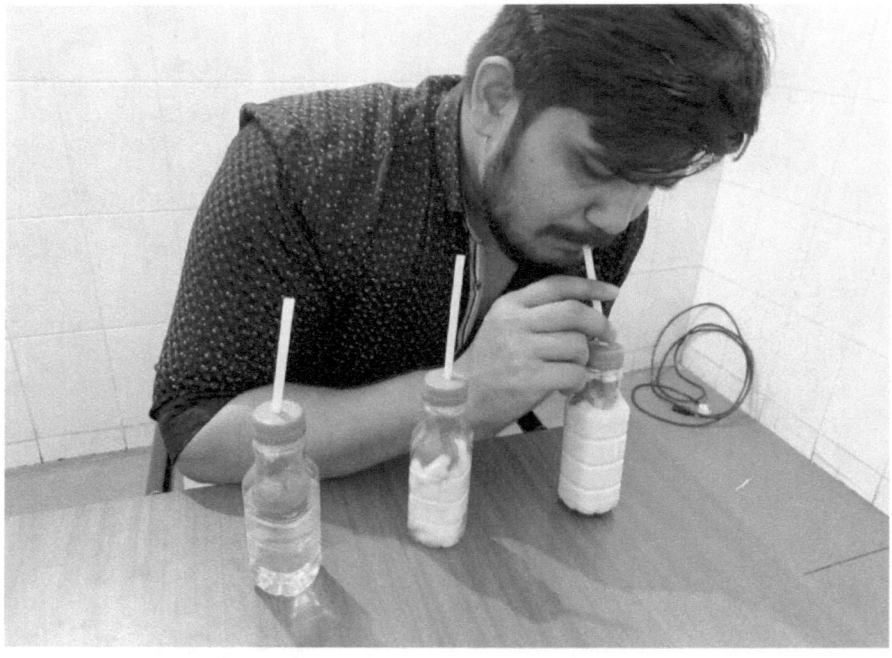

21 | EYE FOR AN EYE

(Is COVID-19 Infliction of Our Own Karma? (The Take-away Message from this Crisis)

Nature has been very lenient on us compared to what we have been doing to it since ages. We have been exploiting it for our selfish intentions. We have been killing animals just to satisfy our cravings and wishes, even though we have the alternative of vegetarian diet.

Law of Retaliation

We have experienced the wrath of the nature from time to time. For every time when the agony reached to its limits, nature has retaliated in vindictive ways. Earthquakes, floods, famines, droughts, epidemics, pandemics etc are the nature "comebacks" to every war inflicted on it by us humans. Every century has witnessed a major disaster which swept substantial population of the world.

What goes Around comes Around!

We cleared huge areas under rainforests for civilization, urbanization etc. We targeted the forests which are called as the "lungs of the earth". Today it's we who are on the receivers end and COVID-19 is thriving in our lungs making us struggle for a single breath of pure oxygen.

We destroyed the natural habitat of various birds, animals, insects, etc. We have taken possession of the lands on which this wild-life had natural claim. They were the true rightful residents of the flora and fauna. But we snatched it from them and today karma has acted and the justice has been served to them. Today we are in hospital beds, immunologically weak succumbed to death beds and animals are wandering freely in our concrete jungles.

We exploited the nature for its natural resources like a bunch of ungrateful's. We never valued what all the nature was bestowing upon us without charging us a single penny. Today, the same ball is in your court. We are getting financially exploited amidst this pandemic, paying double or triple for common commodities.

We polluted water by dumping it with chemicals, waste products, etc damaging the ecosystem for the fishes and other sea creatures, which led to thousands of fishes turning dead floating on the water bodies. Today, it's we humans whose dead bodies are being found bloated, floating on river bodies as the final rites are being denied only on the mere suspicion of being a COVID-19 death.

We rode our bikes and cars in a very ill-judged manner, emitting clouds of black smoke even though we had options of judicious use of the same. We made the air so polluted that today we are forced to wear mask while getting out of our homes. People are being given O_2 through tanks.

A deep breath of pure air is what we are dreaming of in current existing scenario. A tight hug to our closed ones is what is more precious today than lakhs and crores of money. Just to see ourselves without masks is what we crave for ! Things have changed completely and will remain changed forever !

We caged birds against their instincts of flying in the open skies. We petted puppies, kittens, etc against their will. We separated them from their fathers, mothers, brothers, sisters etc. And tadaaa ! Today we are not allowed to be within 1 meter radius of each other. Even a normal hug has been intercepted by the thickness of the PPE kit. There is no face to face communication nowadays. It has been replaced with Mask to Mask formality.

All the above mentioned description has forced our conscience to believe "the vicious cycle of retaliation". It's very rightly said, "Don't worry. Karma always acts. People who hurt you will eventually screw themselves. And if you are lucky enough, god will let you watch." Right now, It's the nature who is sitting on a couch with a bowl of pop-corn and watching the show called "**tragedy of our life**".

Remember, this COVID-19 pandemic is a just a comma and not a full-stop !

22 | TO DO OR NOT TO? – THAT IS THE QUESTION…

Quest for Answer to the Ultimate Survival Dilemma

We are living in such circumstances where in there is a huge disparity between the existence and appearance of various things. Divulgence of statistics reveals that currently in India though the number of cases is attaining a plateau stage, still the balance has been shifted by increased mortality. The number of deaths is exponentially growing resembling a sky-high stack. Every COVID-19 patient has a very unpretentious wish of escaping the death. Every person on ventilator or with NIV mask has a dire desire to just be able to breathe on his own, without any machine or tubes running throughout his body. The big question mark which is still unanswered just keeps on shifting from one subject matter to the other. In a society where the air is filled with fear, stigma, false alarms, disbeliefs, mourns and cries for help; it becomes the moral responsibility of the privileged group to act as the "designated survivors" and stand up to help their falling society rise again.

Amidst the COVID-19 holocaust, number of other potentially life-endangering scenarios are on the verge of outbreak in the near future. The main problem which we are going to face is management of the biomedical wastes. The exponentially accommodating heaps of used masks, syringes, testing kits, body fluid samples etc possess high threat to the society as they might prove to be the starting point of another epidemic.

Second issue is the disposal of bodies of COVID-19 patients. The existing crematoriums have started falling insufficient as a result of the high death rate in India. On top of that the existing stigma related to COVID-19 is only increasing the difficulties especially for the poor people. The question of appropriate disposal of dead bodies is a matter of growing concern nowadays. Reports of dumping dead bodies of COVID-19 patients in rivers are surfacing on a daily basis. The families of the COVID-19 victims have been forced to unwillingly take this step as they were either denied entry to the crematorium or they were financially incapable of bearing the cost for the last rites and had no other option but to leave the bodies of their loved ones in the river.

Third major issue is the "**passively imposed hunger strike**" inflicted upon the daily wage earners. People who have their stomachs supported by their hands have been completely paralyzed since the lockdown. Though the government is trying to revive the financial downfall of this particular sector of the society, still the condition doesn't appear changed. It is the right time for the rich community of the society to give it back to the nation in such critical times when the nation is in desperate need of support. It's not that we can extend our help through financial mode only. Just have a look around your house and whatever you feel is in excess or hasn't been used much, you can donate it to various NGO's and relief-groups which are working day and night to make sure that homeless people get bread and other necessities in this difficult times.

So, the common solution to all the problems mentioned above is "help". Just because you are lucky enough to even survive in this havoc does not mean your free to live inside your little houses. It is your responsibility as a human to make sure that your life gains the necessary meaning by starting to live for others. For the society! For the nation! For our mother earth!

Why to do? Some might ask. It also might erupt in your mind. Because it's this small help which will decide whether you will be "someone" or "no one" for the rest of your lives. It will decide whether you will be able to face yourself in the mirror of conscience towards the end of your lives.

Someone needs oxygen. Someone messages someone. Someone reads the message. Someone amplifies the message. Someone forwards a contact. Someone verifies a contact. Someone answers. Someone collects the cylinder. Someone fills it up. Someone delivers. Someone is saved. All because of someone's will to help someone. So many "someone's" have come forward to serve humanity in these tough times. Be that someone who is restoring faith in humanity by being just someone.

Just by being "someone" opens a lot of doors of possibilities, beliefs, happiness, help and trust. The existence of "someone" is the sign of a thriving society. A society full of "someone's" is what we desperately need right now to overthrow the pessimistic vibes and emerge out of the ashes of destruction just like a Phoenix!

23 | BIBLIOGRAPHY

1. Zhou, B., ThiNhuThao, T., Hoffmann, D. et al. SARS-CoV-2 spike D614G change enhances replication and transmission. *Nature* (2021). https://doi.org/10.1038/s41586-021-03361-1external icon

2. Volz E, Hill V, McCrone J, et al. Evaluating the Effects of SARS-CoV-2 Spike Mutation D614G on Transmissibility and Pathogenicity. Cell 2021; 184(64-75). doi:https://doi.org/10.1016/j.cell.2020.11.020external icon

3. Korber B, Fischer WM, Gnanakaran S, et al. Tracking Changes in SARS-CoV-2 Spike: Evidence that D614G Increases Infectivity of the COVID-19 Virus. Cell 2021; 182(812-7) doi: https://doi.org/10.1016/j.cell.2020.06.043external icon

4. Yurkovetskiy L, Wang X, Pascal KE, et al. Structural and Functional Analysis of the D614G SARS-CoV-2 Spike Protein Variant. Cell 2020; 183(3): 739-751. doi: https://doi.org/10.1016/j.cell.2020.09.032external icon

5. *Davies NG, Abbott S, Barnard RC, et al. Estimated transmissibility and impact of SARS-CoV-2 lineage B.1.1.7 in England. MedRXiv 2021. doi: https://doi.org/10.1101/2020.12.24.20248822external icon

6. Horby P, Huntley C, Davies N et al. NERVTAG note on B.1.1.7 severity. New & Emerging Threats Advisory Group, Jan. 21, 2021. Retrieved from NERVTAG note on variant severityexternal icon

7. Fact Sheet For Health Care Providers Emergency Use Authorization (Eua) Of Bamlanivimab And Etesevimab 02092021 (fda.gov)external icon

8. *Wang P, Nair MS, Liu L, et al. Antibody Resistance of SARS-CoV-2 Variants B.1.351 and B.1.1.7. BioXRiv 2021. doi: https://doi.org/10.1101/2021.01.25.428137external icon

9. *Shen X, Tang H, McDanal C, et al. SARS-CoV-2 variant B.1.1.7 is susceptible to neutralizing antibodies elicited by ancestral Spike vaccines. BioRxiv 2021. doi: https://doi.org/10.1101/2021.01.27.428516external icon

10. *Edara VV, Floyd K, Lai L, et al. Infection and mRNA-1273 vaccine antibodies neutralize SARS-CoV-2 UK variant. MedRxiv 2021. doi: https://doi.org/10.1101/2021.02.02.21250799external icon

11. *Collier DA, DeMarco A, Ferreira I, et al. SARS-CoV-2 B.1.1.7 sensitivity to mRNA vaccine-elicited, convalescent and monoclonal antibodies. MedRxiv 2021. doi: https://doi.org/10.1101/2021.01.19.21249840external icon

12. *Wu K, Werner AP, Moliva JI, et al. mRNA-1273 vaccine induces neutralizing antibodies against spike mutants from global SARS-CoV-2 variants. BioRxiv 2021. doi: https://doi.org/10.1101/2021.01.25.427948external icon

13. Emary KRW, Golubchik T, Aley PK, et al. Efficacy of ChAdOx1 nCoV-19 (AZD1222) Vaccine Against SARS-CoV-2 VOC 202012/01 (B.1.1.7). 2021. The Lancet. doi: http://dx.doi.org/10.2139/ssrn.3779160external icon

14. FACT SHEET FOR HEALTH CARE PROVIDERS EMERGENCY USE AUTHORIZATION (EUA) OF REGEN-COV (fda.gov)external icon

15. *Wang P, Wang M, Yu J, et al. Increased Resistance of SARS-CoV-2 Variant P.1 to Antibody Neutralization. BioRxiv 2021. doi: https://doi.org/10.1101/2021.03.01.433466external icon

16. Pearson CAB, Russell TW, Davies NG, et al. Estimates of severity and transmissibility of novel South Africa SARS-CoV-2 variant 501Y.V2. Retrieved from: pdf (cmmid.github.io) pdficonexternal icon

17. Liu Y, Liu J, Xia H, et al. Neutralizing Activity of BNT162b2-Elicited Serum. 2021. NEJM. DOI: 10.1056/NEJMc2102017

18. *Madhi SA, Ballie V, Cutland CL, et al. Safety and efficacy of the ChAdOx1 nCoV-19 (AZD1222) Covid-19 vaccine against the B.1.351 variant in South Africa. MedRxiv 2021. doi: https://doi.org/10.1101/2021.02.10.21251247external icon

19. Novavax COVID-19 Vaccine Demonstrates 89.3% Efficacy in UK Phase 3 Trial | Novavax Inc. – IR Siteexternal icon

20. Johnson & Johnson COVID-19 Vaccine Authorized by U.S. FDA For Emergency Use | Johnson & Johnson (jnj.com)external icon

21. *Deng X, Garcia-Knight MA, Khalid MM, et al. Transmission, infectivity, and antibody neutralization of an emerging SARS-CoV-2 variant in California carrying a L452R spike protein mutation. MedRxiv 2021. doi: https://doi.org/10.1101/2021.03.07.21252647external icon

22. Xie X, Liu Y, Liu J, et al. SARS-CoV-2 spike E484K mutation reduces antibody neutralisation. The Lancet 2021. doi: https://doi.org/10.1016/S2666-5247(21)00068-9external icon

23. Garcia-Beltran W, Lam EC, St. Denis K, et al. Multiple SARS-CoV-2 variants escape neutralization by vaccine-induced humoral immunity. Cell 2021. doi:https://doi.org/10.1016/j.cell.2021.03.013external icon

24. *Annavajhala MK, Mohri H, Zucker JE, at al. A Novel SARS-CoV-2 Variant of Concern, B.1.526, Identified in New York. MedRxiv 2021. DOI: 10.1101/2021.02.23.21252259external icon

25. *Yadav PD, Sapkal GN, Abraham P, et al. Neutralization of variant under investigation B.1.617 with sera of

BBV152 vaccinees. BioRxiv 2021. DOI: https://doi.org/10.1101/2021.04.23.441101external icon

26. Greaney AJ, Loes AN, Crawford KHD, et al. Comprehensive mapping of mutations in the SARS-CoV-2 receptor-binding domain that affect recognition by polyclonal human plasma antibodies. Cell 2021. DOI: https://doi.org/10.1016/j.chom.2021.02.003external icon

27. *Edara VV, Lai L, Sahoo MK, et al. Infection and vaccine-induced neutralizing antibody responses to the SARS-CoV-2 B.1.617.1 variant. BioRxiv 2021. DOI: https://doi.org/10.1101/2021.05.09.443299external icon

28. https://www.cdc.gov/coronavirus/2019-ncov/variants/variant-info.html

29. https://www.who.int/csr/don/31-december-2020-sars-cov2-variants/en/

30. Rodriguez-Morales AJ, Bonilla-Aldana DK, Balbin-Ramon GJ, Rabaan AA, Sah R, Paniz-Mondolfi A, Pagliano P, Esposito S. 2020. History is repeating itself: Probable zoonotic spillover as the cause of the 2019 novel Coronavirus Epidemic. Infez Med 28(1):3-5.

31. Eastman RT, Roth JS, Brimacombe KR, Simeonov A, Shen M, Patnaik S, Hall MD. Remdesivir: a review of its discovery and development leading to emergency use authorization for treatment of COVID-19. ACS central Science. 2020 May 4;6(5):672-83.

32. Zhou P, Yang XL, Wang XG, et al. A pneumonia outbreak associated with a new coronavirus of probable bat origin. Nature. 2020;579(7798):270–273.

33. Parasher A. Postgrad Med J 2021;**97**:312–320.

34. Zhou P, Yang XL, Wang XG, et al. A pneumonia outbreak associated with a new coronavirus of probable bat origin. Nature. 2020;579(7798):270–273.

35. Warren T, Jordan R, Lo M, et al. Nucleotide prodrug GS-5734 is a broad-spectrumfilovirus inhibitor that provides complete therapeutic protection against the development of Ebola virus disease (EVD) in infected non-human primates. Open Forum Infect Dis. 2015;2(suppl l_1) LB-2.

36. Desforges, M.; Coupanec, A.L.; Dubeau, P.; Bourgouin, A.; Lajoie, L.; Dube, M.; Talbot, P.J. Human coronaviruses and other respiratory viruses: Underestimated opportunistic pathogens of the central nervous system? Viruses **2019**, 12, 14.

37. Mao, L.; Jin, H.;Wang, M.; Hu, Y.; Chen, S.; He, Q.; Chang, J.; Hong, C.; Zhou, Y.;Wang, D.; et al. Neurologic Manifestations ofHospitalized Patients with Coronavirus Disease 2019 in Wuhan, China. JAMA Neurol. **2020**, 77, 683–690.

38. Li, Y.; Li, M.;Wang, M.; Zhou, Y.; Chang, J.; Xian, Y.;Wang, D.; Mao, L.; Jin, H.; Hu, B. Acute cerebrovascular disease followingCOVID-19: A single center, retrospective, observational study. Stroke Vasc. Neurol. **2020**, 5, 279–284.

39. Thakur, V.; Ratho, R.K.; Kumar, P.; Bhatia, S.K.; Bora, I.; Mohi, G.K.; Saxena, S.K; Devi, M.; Yadav, D.; Mehariya, S. Multi-Organ Involvement in COVID-19: Beyond Pulmonary Manifestations. J. Clin. Med. **2021**, 10, 446. https://doi.org/10.3390/jcm10030446

40. Abu Hammad O, Alnazzawi A, Borzangy SS, Abu-Hammad A, Fayad M, Saadaledin S, Abu-Hammad S, Dar Odeh N. Factors influencing global variations in COVID-19 cases and fatalities; a review. InHealthcare 2020 Sep (Vol. 8, No. 3, p. 216). Multidisciplinary Digital Publishing Institute.

41. Ibarrola M, Dávolos I. Myocarditis in athletes after COVID-19 infection: The heart is not the only place to screen. Sports Medicine and Health Science. 2020 Sep 1;2(3):172-3.

42. Guo T, Fan Y, Chen M, et al. Cardiovascular implications of fatal outcomes of patients with coronavirus disease 2019 (COVID-19). JAMA Cardiol. 2020;5(7):1–8 [published

online ahead of print, 2020 Mar 27] https://doi:10.1001/jamacardio.2020.1017.

43. Mujika, I.; Padilla, S. Detraining: Loss of training-induced physiological and performance adaptations. Part II: Long term insufficient training stimulus. Sports Med. **2000**, 30, 145–154.

44. Maron BJ, Udelson JE, Bonow RO, et al; American Heart Association Electrocardiography and Arrhythmias Committee of Council on Clinical Cardiology, Council on Cardiovascular Disease in Young, Council on Cardiovascular and Stroke Nursing, Council on Functional Genomics and Translational Biology, and American College of Cardiology. Eligibility and disqualification recommendations for competitive athletes with cardiovascular abnormalities: task force 3: hypertrophic cardiomyopathy, arrhythmogenic right ventricular cardiomyopathy and other cardiomyopathies, andmyocarditis: a scientific statement from the American Heart Association and American College of Cardiology. *Circulation.* 2015;132(22):e273-e280.

45. Jakobsson J, Malm C, Furberg M, Ekelund U, Svensson M. Physical Activity During the Coronavirus (COVID-19) Pandemic: Prevention of a Decline in Metabolic and Immunological Functions. Frontiers in Sports and Active Living. 2020 Apr 30;2:57.

46. Levine JA. Nonexercise activity thermogenesis–liberating the life-force. Journal of internal medicine. 2007 Sep;262(3):273-87.

47. Levine JA, Schleusner SJ, Jensen MD. Energy expenditure of non exercise activity. Am J ClinNutr 2000; 72: 1451–4.

48. Nardi AE, Cosci F. Expert opinion in anxiety disorder: Corona-phobia, the new face of anxiety. Personalized Medicine in Psychiatry. 2021 Mar 1;25:100070.

49. Postolache TT, Benros ME, Brenner LA. Targetable biological mechanisms implicated in emergent psychiatric conditions associated with SARS-CoV-2 infection. JAMA psychiatry. 2021 Apr 1;78(4):353-4.

50. Rogers JP, Chesney E, Oliver D, Pollak TA, McGuire P, Fusar-Poli P, Zandi MS, Lewis G, David AS. Psychiatric and neuropsychiatric presentations associated with severe coronavirus infections: a systematic review and meta-analysis with comparison to the COVID-19 pandemic. The Lancet Psychiatry. 2020 Jul 1;7(7):611-27.

51. Twenge JM, Joiner TE. US Census Bureau-assessed prevalence of anxiety and depressive symptoms in 2019 and during the 2020 COVID-19 pandemic. Depression and anxiety. 2020 Oct;37(10):954-6.

52. McCann Pineo M, Schwartz RM. Commentary on the coronavirus pandemic: Anticipating a fourth wave in the opioid epidemic. Psychological Trauma: Theory, Research, Practice, and Policy. 2020 Aug;12(S1):S108.

53. Murthy S, Gomersall CD, Fowler RA. Care for critically ill patients with COVID-19. JAMA 2020;323:1499–1500.

54. Baden LR, Rubin EJ. Covid-19—The search for effective therapy. N Engl J Med 2020;382:1787–1799.

55. Chen G, Wu D, Guo W, et al. Clinical and immunological features of severe and moderate coronavirus disease 2019. J Clin Invest May 1 2020;130(5):2620–2629.

56. Wang F, Nie J, Wang H, et al. Characteristics of Peripheral Lymphocyte Subset Alteration in COVID-19 Pneumonia. J Infect Dis May 11 2020;221:1762–1769.

57. CDC COVID-19 Response Team. Preliminary estimates of the prevalence of selected underlying health conditions among patients with coronavirus disease 2019—United States, Centers for Disease Control and Prevention. February 12–March 28, 2020. MMWR Morb Mortal Wkly Rep 2020; 69: 382–86.

58. InstitutoSuperiore di Sanità, COVID-19 Surveillance Group. Characteristics of COVID-19 patients dying in Italy: report based on available data on March 20th, 2020. 2020.

https://www.epicentro.iss.it/coronavirus/bollettino/Report-COVID-2019_20_marzo_eng.pdf. 2020 (accessed June 8, 2020).

59. Guan WJ, Ni Z, Hu Y, et al. Clinical characteristics of coronavirus disease 2019 in China. N Engl J Med 2020; 382: 1708–20.

60. GBD 2017 Disease and Injury Incidence and Prevalence Collaborators. Global, regional, and national incidence, prevalence, and years lived with disability for 354 diseases and injuries for 195 countries and territories, 1990–2017: a systematic analysis for the Global Burden of Disease Study 2017. Lancet 2018; 392: 1789–858

61. Clark A, Jit M, Warren-Gash C, Guthrie B, Wang HH, Mercer SW, Sanderson C, McKee M, Troeger C, Ong KL, Checchi F. Global, regional, and national estimates of the population at increased risk of severe COVID-19 due to underlying health conditions in 2020: a modelling study. The Lancet Global Health. 2020 Aug 1;8(8):e1003-17.

62. Taylor S. The psychology of pandemics: Preparing for the next global outbreak of infectious disease. Cambridge Scholars Publishing; 2019 Oct 7.

63. Nicol GE, Piccirillo JF, Mulsant BH, Lenze EJ. Action at a distance: geriatric research during a pandemic. J Am GeriatrSoc 2020. https://doi.org/10.1111/jgs.16443.

64. Jimenez-Pavon D, Carbonell-Baeza A, Lavie CJ. Physical exercise as therapy to fight against the mental and physical consequences of COVID-19 quarantine: special focus in older people. ProgCardiovasc Dis 2020 Mar 24. https://doi.org/10.1016/j.pcad.2020.03.009.

65. Dubey S, Biswas P, Ghosh R, Chatterjee S, Dubey MJ, Chatterjee S, Lahiri D, Lavie CJ. Psychosocial impact of COVID-19. Diabetes & Metabolic Syndrome: Clinical Research & Reviews. 2020 May 27.

66. Karia, R., Gupta, I., Khandait, H. et al. COVID-19 and its Modes of Transmission. SN Compr.Clin. Med. 2, 1798–1801 (2020)

67. https://www.who.int/emergencies/diseases/novel-coronavirus-2019/advice-for-public

68. Brooks, S. K., Webster, R. K., Smith, L. E., Woodland, L., Wessely, S., Greenberg, N., & Rubin, G. J. (2020). The psychological impact of quarantine and how to reduce it:rapid review of the evidence. Lancet, 395(10227), 912-920.https://doi.org/10.1016/S0140-6736 (20)30460-8.

69. Oronsky B, Larson C, Hammond TC, Oronsky A, Kesari S, Lybeck M, Reid TR. A review of persistent post-COVID syndrome (PPCS). Clinical reviews in allergy & immunology. 2021 Feb 20:1-9.

70. Bone RC (1996) Sir Isaac Newton, sepsis, SIRS, and CARS. Crit Care Med 24:1125–1128

71. Sugimoto MA, Sousa LP, Pinho V, Perretti M, Teixeira MM (2016) Resolution of infammation: what controls its onset?. Front Immunol 7:160. Published 2016 Apr 26

72. Bozza FA, Salluh JI, Japiassu AM, Soares M, Assis EF, Gomes RN, Bozza MT, Castro-Faria-Neto HC, Bozza PT (2007) Cytokine profles as markers of disease severity in sepsis: a multiplex analysis. Crit Care 11(2):R49

73. Delano MJ, Ward PA (2016) The immune system's role in sepsis progression, resolution, and long-term outcome. Immunol Rev 274(1):330–353

74. Kell DB, Pretorius E (2018) To what extent are the terminal stages of sepsis, septic shock, systemic infammatory response syndrome, and multiple organ dysfunction syndrome actually driven by a prion/amyloid form of fbrin?. SeminThrombHemost 44(3):224–238

75. Biradar V, Moran JL (2011) SIRS, Sepsis and Multiorgan Failure. In: Fitridge R, Thompson M, editors. Mechanisms of vascular disease: a reference book for vascular specialists [Internet]. Adelaide (AU): University of Adelaide Press 17. Available from: https://www.ncbi.nlm.nih.gov/books/NBK534275/

76. Hamers L, Kox M, Pickkers P (2015) Sepsis-induced immunoparalysis: mechanisms, markers, and treatment options. Minerva Anestesiol Apr;81(4):426-39. Epub 2014 May 30

77. Dhama, Kuldeep & Khan, Sharun & Tiwari, Ruchi&Sircar, Shubhankar & Bhat, Sudipta & Malik, Yashpal & Singh, Karam & Chaicumpa, Wanpen & Bonilla-Aldana, D. & Rodriguez-Morales, Alfonso. (2020). Coronavirus Disease 2019 – COVID-19. 10.20944/preprints202003.0001.v2.

78. Tipping CJ, Harrold M, Holland A, et al. : The effects of active mobilisation and rehabilitation in ICU on mortality and function: a systematic review. *Intensive Care Med* 2017;43:171–83

www.ingramcontent.com/pod-product-compliance
Lightning Source LLC
Chambersburg PA
CBHW030849180526
45163CB00004B/1510